Heroin Addiction and the British System, Volume II
Treatment and Policy Responses

The 'British System' of dealing with opiate addiction has, for half a century, been notable for its flexibility and its capacity to adapt to changing circumstances. Because of this it has attracted considerable international interest, although it is rarely fully understood or accurately represented.

Presenting a comprehensive account of the development of policies and treatments, *Heroin Addiction and the British System* brings together the perspectives of policy-makers, practitioners, researchers and social commentators. These two volumes contribute to a proper understanding of how policy and practice in the British System have evolved so that lessons for future policy and practice may be identified.

Volume II of *Heroin Addiction and the British System* charts the development and use of such responses in the UK, highlighting the limitations of these approaches as well as their achievements. It is a unique source of reference for students, researchers, healthcare professionals and drug agencies both in the UK and overseas.

Professor John Strang is Director of the National Addiction Centre at the Institute of Psychiatry, King's College London and is Clinical Director of the Addictions Treatment Services for South London and the Maudsley. **Professor Michael Gossop** is a leading researcher at the National Addiction Centre at the Institute of Psychiatry, King's College London and Head of Research, Addictions, at the Maudsley Hospital.

Heroin Addiction and the British System, Volume II

Treatment and Policy Responses

Edited by John Strang and Michael Gossop

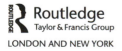
Routledge
Taylor & Francis Group

LONDON AND NEW YORK

First published 2005
by Routledge
2 Park Square, Milton Park, Abingdon, Oxon, OX14 4RN

Simultaneously published in the USA and Canada
by Routledge
270 Madison Ave, New York, NY 10016

Routledge is an imprint of the Taylor & Francis Group

© 2005 John Strang and Michael Gossop, selection and editorial matter;
individual chapters, the contributors

Typeset in Times NR by Graphicraft Limited, Hong Kong
Printed and bound in Great Britain by MPG Books Ltd,
Bodmin, Cornwall

British Library Cataloguing in Publication Data
A catalogue record for this book is available from the British Library

Library of Congress Cataloging in Publication Data
A catalog record has been requested

ISBN 0-415-29816-4 (hbk)
ISBN 0-415-29817-2 (pbk)

Contents

Illustrations

Figures

Tables

Contributors

The editors

John Strang Professor John Strang is Director of the National Addiction Centre (Institute of Psychiatry, King's College London), where he leads the multi-disciplinary treatment and policy research activities and also a Masters degree in the Addictions within the University of London. He is also Clinical Director of the Drug, Alcohol and Smoking Cessation Services of the South London and Maudsley NHS Trust. He was the special consultant advisor on drug treatment services to the Department of Health (England) from 1986 to 2003.

Michael Gossop Professor Michael Gossop is a leading researcher at the National Addiction Centre (Institute of Psychiatry, King's College London), and heads the addictions treatment research at the Maudsley and Bethlem Royal Hospitals. In the mid-1990s, he was responsible for devising and initiating the influential NTORS (National Treatment Outcome Research Study) studying long-term outcome from selected key modalities of treatment in the addictions field.

Chapter authors – Volume II

Mike Ashton Mike Ashton works in an independent freelance capacity and is editor of *Drug and Alcohol Findings*. He previously worked, between 1975 and 1995, at the Institute for the Study of Drug Dependence and was editor of *Druglink*, the house journal of the drugs field in Britain.

Nick Barton Nick Barton trained as a clinical psychologist and is currently Chief Executive of Clouds where he has worked since 1985. Clouds is the registered charity which operates Clouds House, a Twelve-step/abstinence-based programme. He was previously Director of Treatment at Clouds House.

Susan Clement Sue Clement has worked as both a researcher and a clinical psychologist in the addictions field. She was part of an early research study of community alcohol and drugs services in the Manchester region and more widely. She is currently Clinical Senior Lecturer and Honorary Consultant Clinical Psychologist at the University of Hull/Hull and East Riding Community NHS Trust.

Philip Connell Dr Philip Connell was a consultant psychiatrist who established and ran the Drug Dependence Clinical Research and Treatment Unit at the Bethlem Royal and Maudsley Hospitals from 1968 until his retirement in the mid-1980s. He played a key role in the establishment of the British drug clinics during the 1960s and was Chair of ACMD during the important years after the identification of HIV. (Philip Connell died in 1998 at the age of 77 years.)

Michael Farrell Dr Michael Farrell has worked since the early 1990s as a consultant psychiatrist in the South London and Maudsley NHS Trust, and Senior Lecturer at the National Addiction Centre. He has worked as a Policy Advisor to the Department of Health. His research interests include the evaluation of addiction treatment interventions, and studies of psychiatric epidemiology through household surveys.

Emily Finch Dr Emily Finch is a consultant psychiatrist at the South London and Maudsley NHS Trust and Honorary Senior Lecturer at the National Addiction Centre. She has been particularly involved in the establishment of services for drug-misusing offenders, alongside provision of a range of communities addiction treatment services. In 2003, she was also appointed part time to a senior medical position within the National Treatment Agency (NTA).

Philip Fleming Dr Philip Fleming is a consultant psychiatrist in charge of the drug treatment services in Portsmouth, where he has introduced, and given research commentary on, a range of innovative services, including experimental amphetamine maintenance prescribing.

Clare Gerada Dr Clare Gerada is a general practitioner in south London who has championed the enormous potential of interventions in a primary health care setting. As a general practitioner herself, she has demonstrated the potential contribution, as well as leading GP-orientated initiatives such as the new Certificate training in the management of drug misuse within the Royal College of General Practitioners.

Alan Glanz Dr Alan Glanz is a social scientist who has been involved in research study of the addictions field interior settings, including working at the Addiction Research Unit, Institute of Psychiatry, London, during the 1980s. His work has included study of the operation of City Roads, a crisis intervention service in London, and he also conducted the first national survey of GPs and their involvement in treating drug misuse problems. He currently works at the Department of Health.

Laurence Gruer Dr Laurence Gruer is Director of Public Health Science and Information with NHS Health Scotland. He played a central role in planning, building and evaluating a wide range of innovative services for drug users in Glasgow during the 1990s. He has been a member of the Scottish Advisory Committee on Drug Misuse since 1995 and the UK Advisory Council on the Misuse of Drugs (ACMD) since 1996.

Francis Keaney Dr Francis Keaney is a consultant psychiatrist in the addictions. He has worked since 1993 in London drug and alcohol treatment services, and since 1997 at the South London and Maudsley NHS Trust, London. He has conducted research into psychosocial and pharmacological treatments for drug and alcohol dependence.

Tim Leighton Tim Leighton is Head of Professional Education, Training and Research for Clouds, and is a UKCP registered Cognitive Analytical Psychotherapist. He has a particular interest in the role and effectiveness of group therapy.

John Merrill Dr John Merrill is a consultant psychiatrist who has worked in the drug dependence services in Manchester where, through the 1990s, he expanded and consolidated the network of services across the north-west of England. Notwithstanding this expansion, much responsibility still fell to general practitioners – leading to discussion of the relative roles and responsibilities of the specialist and generalist practitioner.

Martin Mitcheson Dr Martin Mitcheson was consultant psychiatrist in charge of the drug dependence unit at University College Hospital in north London, and was an active contributor to the search for a wider range of responses to the diverse drug problems being seen in London at that time. This included close involvement with Phoenix House, and also conduct of the randomised trial of injectable heroin versus oral methadone maintenance. In the mid-1980s, he moved to Bristol where he was instrumental in establishing new regional drug treatment services.

John Polkinghorne The Reverend Dr John Polkinghorne is a physicist and priest who was President of Queen's College Cambridge. In the mid-1990s he was invited to chair of the Government Task Force to Review Services for Drug Misusers, and saw this through to the successful publication of its findings in 1996. He has written books on Quantum Theory, and published many articles.

Duncan Raistrick Dr Duncan Raistrick is a consultant psychiatrist who has led the Leeds Addiction Unit since 1979 where he has been responsible for setting up a wide range of addiction treatment services. He is co-director of a research programme with a special interest in therapist characteristics and treatment outcomes among substance misusers.

Sue Ruben Dr Sue Ruben is Consultant Psychiatrist at the Liverpool Drug Dependency Clinic. She has been lead consultant for drug services in Liverpool since 1988, a time when drug problems were rapidly increasing and when services were still in development. The Liverpool drug services are widely seen as an example of innovative and harm-reduction-oriented service provision.

Janie Sheridan Associate Professor Janie Sheridan is an Addictions researcher with a clinical pharmacy background. Her research work has included investigation of the potential wider role of community pharmacists in the provision of dispensing and harm reduction services for drug misusers. After working for several years as a research worker at the National Addiction Centre, London, she moved to the post of Associate Professor, The School of Pharmacy, Faculty of Medical and Health Sciences, The University of Auckland, New Zealand.

Brian Wells Dr Brian Wells is a consultant psychiatrist who was centrally involved in the establishment of the expanded network of drug treatment services at Charing Cross and elsewhere in north-west London, with managerial as well as clinical involvement. He has also been a long-standing and forthright champion of the important contribution of Narcotics Anonymous (NA) and 12 Step Recovery, and has contributed important personal as well as professional perspectives.

James Willis Dr Jim Willis was Director of the drug clinic at St Giles Hospital in Camberwell, and also consultant psychiatrist at Guy's and Bexley Hospitals, between 1967 and 1976. Thereafter he moved to take up post as the Deputy Medical Director and Head of the Division of Psychiatry at the King Faisal Specialist Hospital Riyadh, Kingdom of Saudi Arabia. He returned to the UK in the mid-1980s and briefly resumed work in the addictions field, before retiring from medical practice and developing a new career as a fiction writer.

John Witton John Witton works as Health Services Research Co-ordinator at the National Addiction Centre, London. Between 1977 and 1997 he was Head of Information Services at the Institute of the Study of Drug Dependence, which served as a focal point for all those involved in the development of drug services and drug policy in Britain at that time.

Deborah Zador Dr Deborah Zador is an Addictions physician, trained in Australia, who has worked in the UK since the late 1990s. She is a Fellow of the Australasian Chapter of Addiction Medicine, Royal Australasian College of Physicians and of the Australasian Faculty of Public Health Medicine. She currently works within the network of Addiction services in Glasgow.

Introduction by the Editors to Volume II

Of all the features of the 'British System', the prescribing of heroin in the name of treatment is the feature that attracts most international fascination – ranging from horror, through intrigue and interest, to adulation. So what are the facts of the history of heroin prescribing in the UK? And how important a position does it occupy in the British System of today? In Chapter 1 to this volume John Strang and colleagues chart the history of the prescribing of heroin and other injectable opiates as part of addiction treatment in the British System up to the present time. (Later in this volume, in Chapter 10, Deborah Zador examines the situation at the beginning of this new century, at a critical point when injectable prescribing has almost disappeared from currently endorsed addiction treatment in the UK.)

One of the defining moments in the construction of a more truly systematic response to drug misuse problems in Britain was the creation of the drug dependence clinics in the late 1960s. Either directly, or indirectly, this laid the foundation for virtually all subsequent responses to the problem. It is surprising, therefore, that the origins of the clinics and the associated thinking have received so little attention. In the next three chapters, the origins and early days of the clinics are described in detail.

Philip Connell was a key figure in the thinking behind the clinics and played a major role in their establishment and early running. In Chapter 2, Connell and Strang describe the emergence of the drug problems in the 1960s, and identification of the need for a more urgent response. The opening of the clinics marked a major change in the relationships which had previously existed between the addict and their doctor, and the chapter plots how the clinics sought to develop a new type of systematic response to the problems of addiction.

Another key player was Jim Willis who, like Philip Connell, was Director of one of the new London clinics. Willis provides a personal view of the behind-the-scenes discussions, arguments and conflicts that surrounded the opening of the clinics. In Chapter 3 Willis offers an insight into some of the developments that have previously remained hidden from view, and their impact on day-to-day life in the new clinics.

Martin Mitcheson was also a Director of one of the London clinics, and in Chapter 4 he moves the discussion forward into the years that followed the initial establishment of the clinics. The 1970s were in many ways a time when the limitations of the clinic system were becoming more apparent. Mitcheson looks at some of the weaknesses and problems which were inherent in that system and at the ways in which the clinics sought to cope with them. The chapter charts some of the problems with staffing, how the clinics coped with the new types of addict and with new types of problems, and the manner in which injectable prescribing fell from favour.

From the earliest days of the clinic system, the demand for treatment began to exceed the capacity of the new services. It became increasingly apparent that a small number of specialist services were not going to be able to meet the demand for treatment. This was undoubtedly one of the reasons for a renewal of interest in the potential contribution of community-based treatment services, including primary health care services.

In Chapter 5, Alan Glanz describes the shifting balance between the specialist and generalist in the treatment of addiction. Part of the reason for the original establishment of the clinics was to remove the treatment of addiction from the GP. Since then there has been a gradual swing back towards the potential contribution of the general practitioner. The role of the GP has more recently been marked by considerable enthusiasm among many of its proponents. An overview of this vision, and the strategy for implementation, is provided in Chapter 6 by Clare Gerada, one of the primary care doctors who has been at the forefront of arguing the case for, and implementing, a major national initiative in primary care. But it is also clear that there have been several problems in translating theory into practice, and, in Chapter 7, John Merrill and Sue Ruben offer a useful critical review of the evidence about how GPs have responded (or not responded) to the challenge of treating people with drug addiction problems.

The introduction of Community Drug Teams across most of the UK during the 1980s and 1990s represented a significant move away from the original specialist clinic system towards a more community-based service which could provide a broader coverage. In Chapter 8, Sue Clement and John Strang describe the thinking behind the development of the Community Drug Teams, and report the early experiences of the CDTs, and also stand back from the venture and reflect on both the achievements and the problems that have been encountered.

Since the early years of the clinics, the prescribing of methadone to outpatients has been at least part of the British System, and since the mid-1970s this has been the most widely used of all the drug treatment options. In Chapter 9, Michael Farrell and Duncan Raistrick present an insight into the manner in which oral methadone maintenance programmes have recently acquired this special status within the UK. This topic is of interest not only because of the central role that this treatment plays within the national treatment system, but also because of the idiosyncracies that exist in the British application of methadone treatment.

In Chapter 10, Deborah Zador looks at the current situation, the crossroads, with regard to heroin prescribing and the other rarer form of methadone prescribing, the provision of injectable methadone. The background to this practice has been covered in Chapter 1. But where has this led the British System? Injectable methadone maintenance is seldom used outside Britain. It has, however, been relatively widely used within the UK, and at a time when there is increasing interest in alternatives to oral methadone maintenance (e.g. heroin maintenance), it is useful to take a closer look at the advantages and disadvantages of methadone when prescribed in its injectable form, alongside the reactivated international interest in heroin maintenance.

For many years, the UK has had an amphetamine misuse problem – rumbling on in the background and occasionally, locally, flaring up into 'epidemics'. However, the treatment of amphetamine misusers has never attracted significant public or professional interest, and there continues to be uncertainty about how amphetamine problems are to be appropriately and effectively treated. One of the contentious options has been that of prescribing amphetamines within a maintenance programme. This is a treatment option that has been used cautiously by Philip Fleming in his drug treatment service on the south coast, and in Chapter 11 he describes the rationale behind this practice and presents the available evidence about its effectiveness.

The impact of HIV/AIDS has been felt throughout addiction treatment services across the world. Within the UK, there was a rapid acknowledgement within the drugs field of the need to respond to these issues at a public health level. In Chapter 12 Janie Sheridan describes how the needle exchange schemes were established and rolled out, both as freestanding services and within pharmacies.

Drug problems can exist as city problems as well as individual problems, as the earlier chapters in Volume I have explored. And so the response can be at the level of the community or city. Laurence Gruer also provides an account of the city-wide public health response to these and related problems. Chapter 13 describes the problems and responses from within one British city (Glasgow). Gruer reports the development of a wave of heroin injecting within the city during the 1980s and how Glasgow created a coordinated city-wide strategy to respond to this problem.

Over the last quarter of the twentieth century, the addiction services within the UK have also been increasingly influenced by a number of treatments which, although they differ in several respects, also share many common features. All owe their origins, to a greater or lesser extent, to Alcoholics Anonymous (AA), and they all share a common focus upon abstinence as the overriding goal of treatment. In Chapter 14, Brian Wells describes the appearance, the growth and the influence of Narcotics Anonymous within

Britain. Brian Wells played an important role within these developments, and his perspective is extremely useful in clarifying these key developments. Following this in the book, although contemporary in time, 12-step residential rehabilitation units were being established. In Chapter 15, Tim Leighton and Nick Barton provide an account of the development of 'Minnesota Model' residential programmes in the UK – from the 1970s onwards. This type of treatment was developed in the United States and has since spread widely and has had a considerable impact upon the way in which residential treatment programmes are designed and delivered. But it has changed in the UK, to become separate from its North American parent, and to become distinctively 'British'.

The issue of 'coerced' treatment has always been a problem for discussion in the addictions. At various times, it has been embraced as an important opportunity or dismissed as unacceptable and ineffective. During the 1990s, many countries, including the UK, have shown an increasing interest in the issue, led primarily by Government departments concerned with crime, not health, leading to major new initiatives. In Chapter 16, Emily Finch and Mike Ashton describe the implementation and impact of the new system of Drug Treatment and Testing Orders which have been introduced within the UK, and also summarise the determination of officials to proceed even in the absence of the proper evidence base.

One of the important events of the 1990s was the establishment of a Government Task Force which was set up to conduct a comprehensive survey of the clinical, operational and cost effectiveness of existing services, and to review current policy in relation to the principal objectives of treatment. This created a considerable stir within treatment services at the time. In Chapter 17, John Polkinghorne, who was chairman of the Task Force, together with Michael Gossop and John Strang, describe the background to the Task Force, how it went about its work, and how the National Treatment Outcome Research Study (NTORS) was commissioned. The chapter describes the immediate and the longer-term impact of NTORS and the Task Force, including some of its unforeseen and unintended consequences.

Finally, in Chapter 18, we have tried to perform an almost impossible editorial task – to bring together the diverse strands and to discern a pattern, a logic or at least an accurate understanding of the important distinctive features that make up the 'British System'. Of course, it is not possible, for there never was a clearly defined or circumscribed 'British System' to describe. Nevertheless, probably as a direct result of this lack of definition, there is an extraordinary richness and diversity to the strands and patterns, many of which have a startling colour or texture not seen in any other country. And this is what has always been, and remains, the enduring fascination of the ever-changing composition which is the 'British System'.

Chapter I

The history of prescribing heroin and other injectable drugs as addiction treatment in the UK

John Strang, Susan Ruben, Michael Farrell, John Witton, Francis Keaney and Michael Gossop

(This chapter draws on a chapter originally published in J. Strang and M. Gossop (eds) *Heroin Addiction and Drug Policy: The British System*, Oxford University Press, 1994.)

Introduction

For years, prescribing injectable heroin to opiate addicts in the name of treatment has been unique to the UK. Indeed, until the mid-1990s, the prescribing of any injectable agonist as part of the treatment for opiate addiction occurred only in the UK, apart from a small scheme with injectable methadone in the Netherlands (Derks 1990), and three patients who represented the rump of 27 heroin addicts who were started on injectable methadone in 1977 in Queensland, Australia (Adrian Reynolds, personal communication, 1993). However, through the late 1990s and early years of the new century, interest in this area has expanded greatly (Bammer *et al.* 1999; Fischer *et al.* 2002). New experimental clinics of supervised injectable heroin prescribing were introduced initially in Switzerland (Perneger *et al.* 1998; Rehm *et al.* 2001; Guttinger *et al.* 2003) and subsequently in the Netherlands (van den Brink *et al.* 2003), prompting consideration of similar new services in other countries also. In addition, there are also a small number of patients on injectable methadone in the east of Switzerland (Stohler *et al.* 1999; Stoermer *et al.* 2003), and a couple of entrenched dependent opiate addicts being treated with injectable methadone in New Zealand (Lee Nixon, personal communication, 2002).

At first glance (and, for some, at second and third glance also) there is something inherently paradoxical in an approach which involves the prescribing of the very drug of addiction as part of the treatment of that addiction. For any consideration of this approach, a particular clarity is required with regard to the goals of treatment. Is it the containment of the 'epidemic' to those already 'infected'? Is it the overcoming of the dependence? Is it the protection from, or muting of, the associated harm? These options will be considered in more detail later in the chapter.

The prescribing of injectable heroin is perhaps the most famous characteristic of the 'British System'. And yet, at the time of writing, it is probably no more than 1 or 2 per cent of the estimated 250,000 heroin users in the UK who receive a prescribed supply of any injectable drug – and only a small proportion of these, probably less than a quarter, will be receiving injectable heroin. In the mid-1990s, the total number of addicts who were receiving a prescribed supply of injectable heroin was estimated from prescription data as approximately three or four hundred (Strang and Sheridan 1999), whilst a further three thousand or so were receiving injectable methadone (Strang *et al.* 1996; Strang and Sheridan 1998). A later report from the same investigators described the steady year-by-year decline in the proportion of NHS methadone prescriptions for injectable versus oral methadone – from 9 per cent of all NHS methadone prescriptions in 1995 down to 3 per cent by 2002 (Strang and Sheridan 2003). For heroin, through their survey of doctors with heroin-prescribing authority, Metrebian *et al.* (2002) identified 448 addict-patients receiving heroin maintenance across the UK. In truth, although this practice may attract considerable local and international attention, the prescribing of injectable drugs in the UK of the late twentieth century was numerically of small significance in the overall UK response – even though the continuity or cessation of the practice may be a subject of great concern to the practitioners and patients for whom it forms the basis of a current treatment.

The guarding of clinical freedom – 'each physician is a law unto himself'

Commentators from abroad, and perhaps especially the USA, are fascinated by the extraordinary clinical freedom which is given to the medical practitioner in the UK with regard to the prescribing of drugs to the opiate addict. As Connell (1975) commented in his review of methadone maintenance schemes, 'each physician in charge of a special drug dependence clinic is a law unto himself as to how he treats and manages patients'. Whilst the prescribing of heroin, cocaine and dipipanone (Diconal) is now restricted to those doctors who hold a special licence (in practice, the doctors who work in National Health Service (NHS) drug treatment centres), any qualified medical practitioner can prescribe oral or injectable methadone, morphine, or any other available pharmaceutical drug. However, despite this extraordinary clinical freedom, the majority of general practitioners choose not to exercise this right so that, paradoxically, the average UK doctor is often extremely conservative in his prescribing to the addict, with three-quarters of a recent national sample of general practitioners reporting that they would not be willing to prescribe oral methadone (Sheridan *et al.*, submitted).

Thus a strange situation has developed, where a small number of general practitioners develop a degree of quasi-specialist expertise in the management of opiate addicts (Gerada *et al.* 2002; see also Chapter 6, this volume), whilst many other general practitioners react hostilely to seemingly modest proposals – such as that they should be involved in the prescribing of oral methadone for at least the purposes of detoxification.

The great variability in prescribing practices results, at least in part, from this lack of central direction. As a result, there is a startling degree of individual clinical freedom for medical practitioners in the UK. For example, there is probably no prescribing whatsoever of any injectable drugs to addicts in the whole of Scotland, Wales, Northern Ireland and much of England, whereas some other areas have NHS drug specialist doctors and other doctors who include the prescribing of injectable heroin or methadone as part of their overall prescribing response. For example, in the national survey of community pharmacists and their dispensing of substitute opiate prescriptions, the proportion of methadone prescriptions in injectable form varied from less than 5 per cent of all methadone prescriptions in several regions up to nearly 25 per cent in one other region (Strang and Sheridan 1998). Whilst the overall number of opiate addicts in a region might obviously vary according to the size of the population and the extent of the local addiction problem, it is hard to believe that such a different proportionate use of injectable maintenance could be explained in this way – as the authors of the study concluded, this seems unlikely to be appropriate tailoring to individuals and is far more likely to be indicative of 'therapeutic anarchy'. This has led to periodic calls for the introduction of new guidelines and new controls: but, meanwhile, the prescription of the injectable drug of main use (or an injectable substitute) continues to exist as a tool within the armamentarium of every doctor in the UK.

The early history of injectable maintenance

In the early twentieth century, the international anti-narcotics movement was becoming influential, and, with the lead taken by the USA, both national and international legislation was passed. After a period during which injectable opiates were prescribed in the USA, the Harrison Act was passed and, after threatened prosecutions to the early maintenance clinics, all prescribing of pharmaceutical opiates to addicts stopped. In contrast, the UK establishment chose not to criminalize but to 'medicalize' the problem, following guidelines from the influential Rolleston Report, which had been prepared as an inter-ministerial report under the chairmanship of Sir Humphrey Rolleston (Ministry of Health 1926; for a fuller account, see Chapter 2 in Volume I by Virginia Berridge). In essence, this report established the right of the medical practitioner in the UK to prescribe regular supplies of an opiate drug to an addict in the following circumstances:

1   where patients are under treatment by the gradual withdrawal method with a view to cure;

2   where it has been demonstrated, after a prolonged attempt to cure, that the use of the drug cannot be safely discontinued entirely on account of the severity of the withdrawal symptoms produced; and

3   where it has been similarly demonstrated that the patient, while capable of leading a useful and normal life when a certain minimum dose is regularly administered, becomes incapable of this when the drug is entirely discontinued.

Thus it was established that the doctor might legally prescribe injectable opiates to an addict provided this was '"treatment" rather than the "gratification of addiction"'.

The next 30 years were a period during which there was no significant problem of injectable opiate use in the UK (also see Chapter 3 in Volume I by Bing Spear). However, although some commentators have eulogized about the effectiveness of the British System during these years, the direction of causality between policy and lack of problem is not clear.

The date when intravenous injecting became established in the UK is not at all clear. The injectable opiate use under consideration by the Rolleston Committee (1926) was subcutaneous or intramuscular, whereas the new opiate injectors in the 1960s (see next section) were mostly using the drug intravenously. In the USA, over this period, there had been a steady spread of the intravenous habit, and this diffusion has been described in some detail (O'Donnell and Jones 1968).

As cracks began to appear in the British System during the 1960s, there was a temptation to look back on what appeared to be the success of the previous decades, identifying characteristics such as the absence of any illicit traffic in drugs, the absence of an addict subculture, and the absence of any young users. However, other commentators suggested that the previous decades had merely been 'a period of non-policy' (Smart 1984) in which 'there was no system, but as there was very little in the way of misuse of drugs, this did not matter' (Bewley 1975). As Downes concluded, the British System had perhaps been 'well and truly exposed as little more than masterly inactivity in the face of what was an almost non-existent addiction problem' (Downes 1977).

Injectable prescribing and the growth of a modern-day problem

In the late 1950s and early 1960s, there was a modest influx of a new type of opiate addict to the UK – a North American (mainly Canadian) addict with an established criminal history. About a hundred such addicts entered the UK during these years, attracted by the accounts of prescribed supplies of injectable pharmaceutical opiates – alongside a lack of immigration restrictions. Some caught the boat to Liverpool and then a train straight to London. For others, the transfer was more direct: 'I got a taxi from the airport to a GP in the Holloway Road, and got an immediate prescription for heroin and cocaine.' (Also see Chapter 3 in Volume I.) Up until this time, the opiate addict population in the UK had been substantially middle-aged and middle-class, with a high representation of doctors and of patients who became dependent on their analgesic drugs. Thus, as a result of the prevailing patterns of prescribing of analgesics, heroin itself was rarely prescribed. For example, during the 1940s and 1950s, the total number of known opiate addicts in the UK never exceeded 500, of whom only about 10 per cent had been using (i.e. were prescribed) heroin.

The interpretation of the events during the 1960s varies greatly, with some observers concluding that the growth of a new drug culture was caused largely by the over-prescribing of a handful of doctors (Second Brain Report (Interdepartmental Committee on Drug Addiction) 1965) whilst others suggest that the lax regulations and generous prescribing potential of UK doctors was a system waiting to be blown open by the newly arrived North American junkies (Blackwell 1988). Whatever the explanation, a youthful hedonistic drug-using culture became established in the UK during the 1960s – particularly in London. The use of injectable opiates involved prescribed pharmaceutical opiates (particularly heroin) which were prescribed by a small number of doctors in or around London, and from whom the daily doses prescribed rose steadily: for example, some of the opiate addicts steadily increased their daily intake from about one to 40 grains of injectable heroin daily (60–2,400 mg daily).

Prescribing injectable drugs from the new clinics (1968 onwards)

NHS drug clinics were established for the first time in 1968. They were expected to address multiple agenda, which included the need to provide treatment to the new addicts, and the need to contain the spreading 'epidemic'. More immediately, there was a need for them to take over the care of more than 1,000 addicts who had been receiving their heroin (and sometimes cocaine) from doctors who were no longer allowed to prescribe either of these two drugs. In practice the majority of these patients were taken on by the clinics on prescriptions very similar to those which they had previously been receiving – at least in the first instance (for further details on the changes at this time, see Chapters 2 and 3, this volume.)

During the early months of operation of the new drug clinics, the new NHS heroin prescribers also took over responsibility for prescribing injectable cocaine – almost exclusively to a population of injecting drug users who were taking both heroin and cocaine. For patients who received both drugs, doses of cocaine were either equal to or lower than the dose of heroin prescribed. However, within a year, an informal agreement was reached amongst London doctors working in the drug clinics to stop the practice of prescribing injectable cocaine: this practice subsequently stopped abruptly for most such patients, since which time only a handful of addicts in the UK have received prescribed supplies of injectable cocaine.

After 18 months of operation, some degree of stability had developed in day-to-day clinic practice. Home Office data are available on the drugs being prescribed to the 1,466 known addicts at the end of December 1969: 499 were receiving prescribed supplies of heroin (of whom 295 were also receiving methadone), 716 were receiving methadone, and 251 were receiving other opiates (usually morphine or pethidine). (Note: most methadone prescribed to addicts in the UK at this time was in the form of injectable methadone ampoules, with only small amounts of oral methadone linctus being prescribed – see Chapters 3 and 4, this volume; however, the exact breakdown of the prescribed drug by route of administration is not provided in the Home Office data.)

Confusion in the clinics:
what purpose is behind injectable prescribing?

During the late 1960s and early 1970s, the new drug doctors (the NHS doctors in the drugs clinics) began to switch their prescribing habits from injectable heroin to injectable methadone (see Chapter 4, this volume). Nevertheless, returns to the Department of Health showed the continued dominance of injectable opiates in the prescriptions to addicts attending NHS hospitals in England and Wales. Examination of the total quantities of injectable heroin, injectable methadone and oral methadone (the three main forms of opiates prescribed to addicts) prescribed reveals a gradual change during the decade after the opening of the clinics, with annual figures of 17, 11 and 3 kg, respectively, being prescribed in 1970; 15, 21 and 8 kg, respectively, in 1974; and 9, 14 and 17 kg respectively, by 1978 (Department of Health data published by Edwards 1981).

Prescription of injectable methadone steadily increased to a mid-1970s peak, after which the trend appears to have been away from any injectable prescribing, with an increased reliance on oral methadone. These data accord with the findings of Blumberg *et al.* (1974) who reported on the slightly greater obtainability of injectable methadone than injectable heroin in the early 1970s. It is also interesting to note from Blumberg's work that injectable methadone and heroin are accorded similar scores by the addict for liking and need.

This potential conflict was explored by Stimson and Oppenheimer (1982). If clinicians were to be expected to walk a 'prescribing tightrope' and if clinics were to be given the twin aims of medical care and social control, could these aims always be met together, or might they sometimes be in conflict? As they illustrated, 'for example, the social control of addiction might be best pursued by a maintenance-prescribing approach, but this might not be the best treatment for an individual patient . . .'. At the end of the day, for society at large, even if not for the clinicians, the social control of addiction was usually seen as the primary task of the clinics.

This conflict was also considered by Mitcheson and Hartnoll in one of the early considerations of their study of prescribing injectable heroin versus oral methadone. They observed that

> overall, prescribing heroin can be seen as maintaining the status quo with the majority of heroin-maintained patients continuing to inject heroin regularly: prescribing heroin is not associated with an improvement in social functioning or a reduction in consumption of illegal drugs, as is sometimes claimed. It may reduce the degree of involvement in criminal activity, especially in terms of arrests and conviction rates. Refusal to prescribe heroin, while offering oral methadone, constitutes a more confrontational response by the clinic and results in a higher abstinence rate. On the other hand this treatment is less acceptable to the client and the clinic fails to maintain a regular contact with the group of clients who continue to use illicit drugs. . . .
>
> (Mitcheson and Hartnoll 1978)

What was behind the move from prescribing injectable heroin to prescribing injectable methadone? No doubt it was partly influenced by the increased public and professional anxiety about prescribing heroin (in the public's eyes, a drug of abuse) compared with methadone (in public and professional eyes, a medicinal drug). However, other reasons were also articulated. The long half-life of methadone meant that it might be a drug which was more conducive to social and occupational stability, as it need only be administered once or twice a day.

There were also concerns about the safety of injecting heroin: pharmaceutical heroin was prescribed in the 1960s and 1970s in the form of tablets known as pills or jacks, which the addict (or nurse or doctor) would then dissolve in water to make the solution ready for injecting. As Bewley said,

> we tend to prescribe methadone because it comes in an ampoule and it won't be mixed with water from the kitchen sink or whatever: also because it's a more long-acting drug. There is no evidence that it is better than heroin in one way or another but because it is more long-acting and because people can inject it in a cleaner way, we believe that there is an advantage.
>
> (Bewley 1975)

Injectable heroin and injectable methadone

Methadone has a hedonistic appeal and black market value which is similar to heroin when both drugs are compared in their injectable forms (see Blumberg et al. 1974). Internationally, methadone is often considered only in its oral form, and observers mistakenly attribute properties to the drug itself when they are in fact confusing the drug with the formulation. Only recently has serious attention to injectable methadone maintenance been included in guidance and text books about methadone treatment (e.g. Tober and Strang 2003). In clinical practice with the prescribing of these drugs to opiate addicts, the committed injector seeking a prescribed supply of inject-able drugs would usually be quite amenable to moves between heroin and methadone in injectable form – in sharp contrast to the determined opposi-tion which may be encountered to suggestions of moving from injectable methadone to its oral form. In an interview with one such addict receiving injectable methadone in Amsterdam, the addict is quoted as follows: 'I have been taking it for half a year now, it's far out: they can take anything from me, my beer, my wife – so long as they keep their hands off my injectable methadone' (Kools 1992).

Not just the opiates

The debate about prescribing of injectable drugs to addicts is usually dominated by consideration of prescribing opiate drugs. However, other drugs of dependence have also been prescribed in injectable forms, although this practice has become extremely rare.

When the new NHS drug clinics were established in 1968, many of the patients who were taken on from the private practitioners were already receiving prescribed supplies of intravenous cocaine alongside their prescribed intravenous heroin. Initially the doctors in the new drug clinics continued this prescribing of cocaine – up until a consensus was reached amongst these doctors to cease all such cocaine prescribing (in late 1968), which appears to have been implemented extensively with little or no evidence of the promotion of a rebound black market in imported cocaine. A small number of doctors continued to prescribe injectable cocaine to extremely small numbers of addict patients (usually in conjunction with injectable opiates), but only a handful of such cases continued through to the 1980s.

An intravenous methylamphetamine epidemic occurred during 1967/68, when a small number of private doctors (whom the new regulations banned from prescribing heroin or cocaine) began to prescribe methylamphetamine ampoules (Methedrine) with a resulting epidemic of chaotic use (James 1968; Hawks et al. 1969). One London centre began an experimental programme of prescribing injectable amphetamines to these drug users, but this was soon abandoned when an agreement was reached between the Ministry of Health and the manufacturers to withdraw supplies of methylamphetamine to retail chemists (hence closing off its availability via private doctors) (Mitcheson *et al.* 1976).

Whilst the interruption of cocaine prescribing (see previous paragraph) might have been linked to the development of this methylamphetamine abuse (in that the methylamphetamine was being prescribed by many of the same private doctors who were no longer able to prescribe cocaine), the co-ordinated control strategy of removal of supplies of the drug from retail pharmacists would appear to stand as an example of a successful control-based intervention.

AIDS breathes new life into the injectable prescribing debate

The debate about the appropriateness or otherwise of prescribing injectable drugs continued as a background debate during the early 1980s, but shifted from being a debate within specialist clinic practice to being the battleground between NHS and private doctors. However, it remained an extremely rare form of clinical practice in most areas, so that by the mid- to late 1980s there were probably still only a couple of thousand addicts in receipt of injectable drugs (mainly injectable methadone) from amongst the estimated 75,000–150,000 opiate addicts (Advisory Council on the Misuse of Drugs (ACMD) 1988).

Acquired immune deficiency syndrome (AIDS) brought a fundamental re-examination of drug policy and the goals and methods of drug treatment in the UK (ACMD 1988, 1989; Strang and Stimson 1990; Department of Health 1991). The prescribing of injectable drugs was back on the main agenda – not necessarily as a recommended practice, but certainly as an option to be considered. Prescribing of any drugs to the drug user was reformulated as a possible 'useful tool in helping to change the behaviour of some drug misusers either towards abstinence or towards intermediate goals such as a reduction in injecting or sharing' (ACMD 1988). A hierarchy of acceptable goals was identified:

1   the cessation of sharing of equipment;
2   the move from injectable to oral drug use;
3   a decrease in drug use; and
4   abstinence.

For this consideration, any prescribing could be judged and compared according to its effectiveness/ineffectiveness in bringing about the desired changes. The prescribing of injectable drugs was included in this consideration, but with the caveat that such cases should not be managed by the general practitioner and required input from specialist drug services. The ACMD (1988) went on to state that in some cases – a small minority – there may be a need initially to prescribe injectable drugs to ease the change from injecting the drug of dependence to taking a substitute orally, but that there is a substantial risk that these injectable drugs will be abused in addition to other drugs and that the injectable prescribing may perpetuate and aggravate the injecting addiction problem. Consequently they recommended that such cases should be seen more frequently and should be managed by, or with guidance from, the District or Regional specialist team.

Thus the ACMD endorsed the view that interim prescribing of injectable drugs might be considered legitimate medical practice if it was found to bring about a move that was ultimately towards oral-only use which might otherwise not have occurred: in these circumstances, the end would have justified the means.

Nevertheless, despite all the discussion about the possible special role for injectable prescribing, no funding ever emerged for serious research study of this new use of injectable prescribing and, in this research vacuum, professional and public argument continued – with a characteristic excess of heat over light. Injectable prescribing continued to exist, but only in a haphazard manner according to the whim or personal passion of the local individual specialist, which presumably partly accounts for the regional variation described above. And so it was this debate ultimately failed to be translated into widespread practice – not so much because the scientific evidence was against it, but more because it continued to be just debate and conjecture, without any research evidence base to which reference could be made.

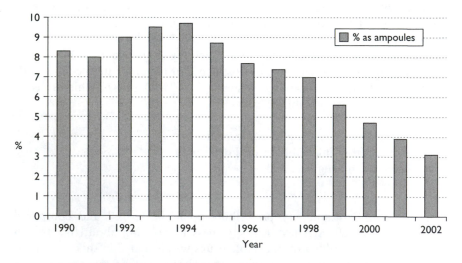

Figure 1.1 Changing proportion of NHS methadone prescriptions in ampoule form, England 1990–2002

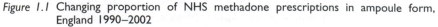

Source: Derived from Department of Health statistical reports.

Some tangible evidence of the dwindling role of injectable maintenance can be seen by looking at Department of Health national data on methadone prescribing, which report separately on the prescriptions according to their different formulations, thereby enabling calculation of the annual proportion of all methadone prescriptions issued as either oral or injectable methadone. This is shown in Figure 1.1, from which it can be seen that injectable methadone maintenance has steadily reduced from a level of about 10 per cent of all methadone prescriptions in the mid-1990s to a much lower level of only 5 per cent by the end of the 1990s and only 3 per cent by 2002 (Strang and Sheridan 2003).

Switzerland and the Netherlands prompt new British self-examination of injectable maintenance

In the early 1990s, Switzerland was experiencing a major heroin problem which included, in cities such as Zurich, a distinctive feature of large numbers of heroin users putting themselves at risk and creating a public nuisance by gathering in major parks and other such public places. As part of their response, the Swiss introduced a variant of the 'British System' of heroin prescribing, which they adapted so as to be greatly more efficient and disciplined in the organization and provision of the heroin maintenance. In total, nearly 2,000 addicts were started on heroin maintenance at more than 20 centres across the country, with the heroin addict attending the clinic, usually several times per day, to take their heroin under supervision – thereby avoiding concerns about diversion of the prescribed heroin onto the black market and the consequent overdose risk.

In the late 1990s, following reports of the success of the Swiss 'experiment', a more controlled heroin trial was established in the Netherlands, involving more than 500 addicts across six centres, with patients randomly allocated to the standard treatment of oral methadone or to the experimental treatment of heroin (as either injectable heroin or in smokable form). Here again, the patient attended the clinic several times per day in order to self-administer their heroin under supervision, thereby avoiding risks of feeding a black market and contributing to the wider community overdose risk. In the Dutch trial, the patients who received either injectable or smokable heroin did better than those treated with methadone alone on most measures of outcome, including improvements in physical health, mental status and social functioning (van den Brink *et al.* 2003). One exception to this was for treatment retention. Perhaps somewhat surprisingly, retention rates after 12 months were higher among the methadone-only group (86%) than among those receiving heroin (70%). Considering that patients were chronic, non-responders to methadone maintenance treatment, another interesting if unexpected finding was the relatively high rate of clinical improvement among patients in the control groups who continued to receive methadone.

The debate continues about the conclusions that can be reached from these two national 'experiments'. But one thing is certain. These developments stimulated a new public interest and international political debate about the contributions of heroin prescribing, thereby re-activating consideration within the UK about a possible rebirth of the 'British System'.

Concern about drug-related crime unexpectedly stimulates re-examination of injectable maintenance

In the absence of a research evidence base, a topic such as heroin prescribing is particularly likely to be influenced by political disapproval or favour. To considerable public and professional surprise, David Blunkett, who was appointed in 2001 as the new Home Secretary, took hold of the reins of British drug policy, displaced the UK 'drugs Tsar', and began to brief journalists about his wish for a radical re-think of British drug policy. One of the areas that understandably concerned him was the substantial contribution to property crime which was partly a result of the steadily growing problem of heroin addiction. And one of the solutions that he wished to be considered was the possibly much wider provision of heroin maintenance, in the way he had heard described as being so effective in Switzerland and the Netherlands. Prompted partly by this senior ministerial interest, the House of Commons Home Affairs Committee subsequently considered this area and made several recommendations which supported the serious consideration of wider provision of injectable heroin maintenance (House of Commons, 2002).

The distinctive new feature about this support for injectable maintenance is the source and nature of the pressure – it is a pressure from the criminal justice system, and it is a pressure for a treatment that is primarily concerned with the extent of associated crime. Earlier versions of injectable heroin prescribing in the British System have been driven by a more orthodox health orientation, with the treatment being conceptualized within a medical framework of treatment for individuals with an addiction disorder. But the new concern was that 'on some estimates, one third of all property crime in the UK is judged to be drug-related' (House of Commons, 2002) and there was an endorsement of reduction of drug-related anti-social and criminal behaviour as a major aim of the Government's drug strategy, alongside (in fact preceding) the aim of providing treatment to those suffering drug problems. With evident reliance on the evidence presented about the Swiss and Dutch heroin prescribing, the Home Affairs Select Committee recommended a substantial increase in the extent of heroin prescribing, whilst also recommending that this should be 'targeted, in the first instance, at chronic addicts who were prolific offenders'.

Concluding observations

Doctors as healers, or doctors as grocers?

The introduction and spread of needle-exchange schemes in the UK since 1987 (Stimson *et al.* 1988, 1990) represented not only a new service to the actual or potential clientele of the drug clinics, but also provoked a widening of the constituency of concern. The needle-exchange schemes not only provide needles and syringes to the established addict (who may or may not be known to drug treatment services), but also to the non-dependent injector. What should be the response of drug treatment services to the non-dependent injector? On the one hand, it could be argued that the next logical step is to provide free supplies of the pharmaceutical drugs to put into the free needles and syringes, whilst on the other hand this could be seen as a naive and ill-considered position which fails to appreciate the fundamentally different nature of the strategies behind drug treatment services and needle and syringe services.

Should the doctor prescribe the drugs to fit inside the needle and syringe – and for the non-dependent user as well as for the addict? If they were to do so, it could be argued that the doctor is no longer providing medical treatment to the individual, but is now little more than an overpaid grocer whose only task is to provide the products as requested (perhaps with some safety cut-off limits). Self (1995) has described this as doctors acting as 'dealers by appointment to H.M. Government'. This confusion between the availability of drugs as treatment and the availability of drugs as commodities is evident in some of the calls for legalization of drugs, where many of the points made relate to the provision of treatment to addicts (and could hence be considered in a different context). At the end of the day, the debate is essentially about the legitimate purpose behind the doctor (or other health-care worker) providing drugs to the drug addict, and about different legitimizing ideologies behind the provision of drugs to drug users.

Is there a future for injectable opiate maintenance in the UK?

The option of prescribing heroin and other injectable drugs has long been a distinctive feature of the British System. Consequently it should prompt great collective shame and national embarrassment that the UK is still unable to answer even the simplest questions about the research evidence base for this controversial practice. The failure to invest in the necessary studies to get good scientific answers to the most basic of questions means that the field remains extremely vulnerable to public prejudice and political whim. As a result, no reliable conclusions can be reached about injectable maintenance on the basis of UK evidence, leaving the issue wide open to hijack by those who wish to reinforce their already-formed positions within the prescribing debate.

The current situation, and the implications for the future for injectable opiate maintenance, are considered in more detail in Chapter 10, this volume.

References

ACMD (Advisory Council on the Misuse of Drugs) (1988). AIDS and drug misuse report. Part 1. HMSO, London.

ACMD (1989). AIDS and drug misuse report. Part 2. HMSO, London.

ACMD (1993). AIDS and drug misuse report. Update. HMSO, London.

Bammer, G., Dobler-Mikola, A., Fleming, P., Strang, J. and Uchtenhagen, A. (1999). The heroin prescribing debate: integrating science and politics. *Science*, 284: 1277–8.

Banks, A. and Waller, T. A. N. (1988). *Drug misuse – a practical handbook for GPs.* Blackwell Scientific Publications, Oxford.

Battersby, M., Farrell, M., Gossop, M., Robson, P. and Strang, J. (1992). 'Horsetrading': prescribing injectable opiates to opiate addicts. A descriptive study. *Drug and Alcohol Review*, 11, 35–42.

Bewley, T. H. (1975). Evaluation of addiction treatment in England. In *Drug dependence: treatment and treatment evaluation* (ed. H. Bostrom, T. Larsson and N. Ljungstedt), pp. 275–86. Almquist & Wiksell, Stockholm.

Blackwell, J. (1988). The saboteurs of Britain's opiate policy: over-prescribing physicians or American-style junkies? *International Journal of the Addictions*, 23, 517–26.

Blumberg, H., Cohen, S., Dronfield, B., Mardecai, E., Roberts, J. and Hawks, D. (1974). British opiate users: I. People approaching London drug treatment centres. *International Journal of the Addictions*, 9, 1–23.

Connell, P. H. (1975). Review of methadone maintenance schemes. In *Drug dependence – treatment and treatment evaluation* (ed. H. Bostrom, T. Larsson and N. Ljundstedt), pp. 133–46. Almquist & Wiksell, Stockholm.

Dally, A. (1990). *A doctor's story.* Macmillan, London.

Department of Health and Social Security (1984). Guidelines for good clinical practice in the treatment of drug misuse. DHSS, London.

Department of Health, Scottish Home and Health Department, and Welsh Office (1991). Drug misuse and dependence: guidelines on clinical management, pp. 35–6. HMSO, London.

Derks, J. (1990). The efficacy of the Amsterdam morphine-dispensing programme. In *Drug misuse and dependence* (ed. A. H. Ghodse, C. Kaplan and R. Mann), pp. 85–108. Parthenon, Carnforth.

Downes, D. (1977). The drug addict as folk devil. In *Drugs and politics* (ed. P. Rock), pp. 89–97. Transaction Books, New Jersey.

Edwards, G. (1981). The Home Office Index as a basic monitoring system. In *Drug problems in Britain: a review of ten years* (ed. G. Edwards and C. Busch), pp. 25–50. Academic Press, London.

Fischer, B., Rehm, J., Kirst, M., Hall, W., Krausz, M., Metribian, N., Reggers, J., Uchtenhagen, A., van den Brink, W. & van Ree, J. M. (2002). Heroin-assisted treatment as a response to the public health problem of opiate dependence. *European Journal of Public Health*, 12: 228–34.

Gerada, C. and Murnane, M. (2003). Royal College of General Practitioners' Certificate in Drug Misuse. *Drugs: Education, Prevention and Policy*, 10: 369–79.

Ghodse, A. H. (1992). Care of addicts in police custody. *The Times*, 25 February, p. 11.

Glanz, A., Byrne, C. and Jackson, P. (1989). Role of community pharmacies in prevention of AIDS among injecting drug misusers: findings of a survey in England and Wales. *British Medical Journal*, 209, 1076–9.

Guttinger, F., Gschwend, P., Schulte, B., Rehm, J., Uchtenhagen, A. (2003). Evaluating long-term effects of heroin-assisted treatment: the results of a 6-year follow-up. *European Addiction Research*, 9: 73–9.

Hawks, D. V., Mitcheson, M., Ogborne, A. and Edwards, G. (1969). Abuse of methylamphetamine. *British Medical Journal*, 2, 715–21.

House of Commons (2002). *The Government's drug policy: is it working?* The Stationery Office, London.

Interdepartmental Committee on Drug Addiction (Brain Committee) (1965). Drug addiction; second report. HMSO, London.

James, I. P. (1968). A methylamphetamine epidemic. *Lancet*, i, 916.

Kools, J. P. (1992). Injectable methadone: policy for supplying methadone. *Mainline: Drugs, Health and the Street* (special edition), p. 5.

Metrebian, N., Carnwath, T., Stimson, G. and Storz, T. (2002). Survey of doctors prescribing diamorphine (heroin) to opiate-dependent drug users in the United Kingdom. *Addiction*, 97, 1155–61.

Ministry of Health (1926). Report of the Departmental Committee on Morphine and Heroin Addiction (Rolleston Report). HMSO, London.

Mitcheson, M. and Hartnoll, R. (1978). Conflicts in deciding treatments within drug dependency units. In *Problems of drug abuse in Britain* (ed. D. J. West), pp. 74–9. Institute of Criminology, Cambridge.

Mitcheson, M., Edwards, G., Hawks, D. and Ogborne, A. (1976). Treatment of methylamphetamine users during the 1968 epidemic. In *Drugs and drug dependence* (ed. G. Edwards, M. Russell, D. Hawks and M. MacCafferty), pp. 155–62. Saxon House, Farnborough.

O'Donnell, J. A. and Jones, J. D. (1968). Diffusion of the intravenous technique among narcotic addicts. *Journal of Health and Social Behaviour*, 9, 120–30.

Perneger, T. V., Giner, F., del Rio M. and Mino, A. (1998). Randomised trial of heroin maintenance programme for addicts who fail in coinventional drug treatments. *British Medical Journal*, 317: 13–18.

Rehm, J., Gschwend, P., Steffen, T., Gutzwiller, F., Dobler-Mikola, A., & Uchtenhagen, A. (2001). Feasibility, safety and efficacy of injectable heroin prescription for refractory opioid addicts: a follow-up study. *Lancet*, 358: 1417–23.

Robertson, R. (1987). *Heroin, AIDS and society*. Hodder & Stoughton, London.

Self, W. (1995). Drug dealer by appointment to H.M. Government. In *Junk Mail*, pp. 83–91. Penguin: London.

Smart, C. (1984). Social policy and drug addiction: a critical study of policy development. *British Journal of Addiction*, 79, 31–9.

Stimson, G. V. (1973). *Heroin and behaviour: diversity among addicts attending London clinics*. Irish University Press, Shannon.

Stimson, G. V. and Oppenheimer, E. (1982). *Heroin addiction: treatment and control in Britain*. Tavistock, London.

Stimson, G., Alldritt, L., Dolan, K. and Donoghoe, M. (1988). Syringe exchange schemes for drug users in England and Scotland. *British Medical Journal*, 296, 1717–19.

Stimson, G., Donoghoe, M., Lart, R. and Dolan, K. (1990). Distributing sterile needles and syringes to people who inject drugs: the syringe exchange experiment. In *AIDS and drug misuse: the challenge for policy and practice in the 1990s* (ed. J. Strang and G. Stimson), pp. 222–31. Routledge, London.

Stoermer, R., Drewe, J., Dursteler-MacFarland, K. M., Hock, C., Mueller-Spahn, F., Ladewig, D., Stohler, R. and Mager, R. (2003). Safety of injectable opioid maintenance treatment for heroin dependence. *Biological Psychiatry*, 54: 854–61.

Stohler, R., Dursteler, K. M., Stoermer, R., Seifritz, E., Hug, I., Sattler-Mayr, J., Muller-Spahn, F., Ladewig, D. and Hock, C. (1999). Rapid cortical hemoglobin deoxygenation after heroin and methadone injection in humans: a preliminary report. *Drug and Alcohol Dependence*, 57: 23–8.

Strang, J. (1990). The roles of prescribing. In *AIDS and drug misuse: the challenge for policy and practice in the 1990s* (ed. J. Strang and G. Stimson), pp. 142–52. Routledge, London.

Strang, J. (1992). Harm reduction for drug users: exploring the dimensions of harm, their measurement and the strategies for reduction. *AIDS and Public Policy Journal*, 7(3), 145–52.

Strang, J. (1993). Drug use and harm reduction: responding to the challenge. In *Harm reduction: from faith to science* (ed. N. Heather, A. Wodak, E. Nadelman and P. O'Hare), pp. 3–20. Whurr Publishers, London.

Strang, J. and Gossop, M. (eds) (1994). *Heroin addiction and drug policy: the British system*. Oxford University Press, Oxford.

Strang, J. and Sheridan, J. (1997). Heroin prescribing in the 'British System' of the mid 1990s: data from the 1995 national survey of community pharmacies in England and Wales. *Drug and Alcohol Review*, 16: 7–16.

Strang, J. and Sheridan, J. (1998). National and regional characteristics of methadone prescribing in England and Wales: local analyses of data from the 1995 national survey of community pharmacies. *Journal of Substance Misuse*, 3: 240–6.

Strang, J. and Sheridan, J. (2003). Injectable methadone prescribing: a peculiarly British treatment. In *Methadone matters – evolving community methadone treatment of opiate addiction* (ed. G. Tober and J. Strang), pp. 91–105. Dunitz, London.

Strang, J. and Stimson, G. (1990). The impacts of HIV: forcing the process of change. In *AIDS and drug misuse: the challenge for policy and practice in the 1990s* (ed. J. Strang and G. Stimson), pp. 3–15. Routledge, London.

Strang, J., Sheridan, J., Barber, N. and Glanz, A. (1996). Role of community pharmacies in relation to HIV prevention and drug misuse: findings from the 1995 national survey in England and Wales. *British Medical Journal*, 313: 272–4.

Tober, G. and Strang, J. (eds) (2003). *Methadone matters – evolving community methadone treatment of opiate addiction*. Dunitz, London.

Van den Brink, W., Hendriks, V. M., Blanken, P., Koeter, M. W., van Zwieten, B. J., and van Ree, J. M. (2003). Medical prescription of heroin to treatment resistant heroin addicts: two randomized controlled trials. *British Medical Journal*, 327: 310.

Chapter 2

The origins of the new drug clinics of the 1960s

Clinical demand and the formation of policy

Philip Connell and John Strang

(This chapter originally appeared in J. Strang and M. Gossop (eds) *Heroin Addiction and Drug Policy: The British System*, Oxford University Press, 1994.)

The 1960s were a time of great social upheaval and change – particularly amongst the newly-emergent youth culture and their relationship with the establishment. Their iconoclasm found expression in various ways including, for some groups, the use of illicit drugs. In some ways this drug use can be seen as paralleling the search for new identities, new ways of living, and the search for chemical shortcuts to higher planes of enjoyment and self-discovery. But it was not just the significance of the drug use which was changing – major changes occurred in the substances being used, in the manner in which they were being used, and in the characteristics of the drug takers themselves.

For several decades up to the 1950s, the UK drug problem had been notable by its absence (see Chapters 2 and 3, Volume I), and a similar picture was seen across Europe – in contrast to the situation in the USA. No significant drug problem existed to test the adequacy or appropriateness of UK drug policy, and no significant clinical demand existed to test the adequacy and appropriateness of the treatment response. Perhaps the most clear demonstration of these changes is evident by looking at the ages of addicts in the UK. As Spear has described (1969; see also Chapter 3, Volume I), the number of opiate addicts in the UK had been fairly constant between 400 and 600 during any year, of whom half were deemed to be therapeutic addicts who had become addicted to the drug during the course of treatment for pain associated with a physical disorder. A substantial number of the remainder were physicians or other professionals who had unusual access to pharmaceutical supplies of the drug. Of this number there were less than a hundred who were addicted to heroin, and these addicts were nearly all middle-aged or older. Indeed the first known case of a heroin addict under the age of 20 years was not until 1960. Yet by 1967 there were

381 known cases of heroin addiction who were aged less than 20 years, and 827 aged between 20 and 34 years, and the annual numbers of heroin addicts had increased from about 50 to a 1967 figure of 1,299.

This chapter is a synthesis of various perspectives given at the time of the creation of the clinics in 1968. New perspectives were emerging on the phenomenon itself, new services were being created, and new methods of dealing with the problem of drug dependence were starting. A new analysis was evidently required.

The new analysis

The first report from the Brain Committee (Interdepartmental Committee) had appeared in 1961 and was generally reassuring – the drug problem was small, static, and no special measures needed to be taken; it was predominantly a medical, not a criminal, problem. However, in view of the changes of the early/mid-1960s, the Committee was hastily reconvened in 1964 and published its influential Second Report (Interdepartmental Report 1965). The phenomenon itself (drug use) was seen as socially infectious, and indeed various studies of heroin use traced the chain of transmission of local spread by peer group 'infection' (de Alarcon and Rathod 1968; Kosviner et al. 1968; de Alarcon 1969). Sweeping recommendations were made by the Second Brain Committee: these recommendations stand as the output of a major new reconsideration of the UK drug problem, which had continued largely unaltered (and indeed largely unchallenged) since the Rolleston Report (1926; see Chapter 2, Volume I). Thus the Second Report of the Brain Committee recommended: the introduction of limits on the rights of doctors to prescribe heroin or cocaine (so that only those doctors holding a special licence could prescribe either of these drugs to addicts); the setting up of specialist out-patient clinics with back-up in-patient provision (especially in London); the introduction of compulsory notification of addiction (along the lines of infectious diseases notification, but managed by the Home Office); encouragement of research into drug addiction; and the creation of a Standing Advisory Committee to look over developments in the problem and the response.

The pace of change at the time was such that urgent action was required. Over the course of four years (1964–68), UK policy and practice moved from an unspecified and individually determined response to less than a hundred heroin addicts in 1964 through to a network of specialist drug treatment clinics (mainly in the London area) as part of mental health services for about 2,000 heroin addicts. By 1961, Frankau and Stanwell were, for the first time, able to describe extensive experience of private treatment of heroin addicts, some of whom had recently arrived from Canada (see Zacune 1971), and some of whom were an indigenous population (Frankau and Stanwell 1961); and by 1964 Hewettson and Ollendorf were able to describe their general practitioner (GP) experience of 100 heroin addicts in south London (Hewettson and Ollendorf 1964). And yet the majority of the medical profession was not involved and did not wish to be involved. In the words of one GP active in the drug field, the proposal for new services 'was flying in the face of established medical opinion in this country, which regards the prescribing of narcotic drugs as incorrect for the treatment of addiction. This dilemma is still present – namely that the majority of doctors question prescribing as a policy in this treatment' (Chapple 1967).

The pace of contemporary debate was fast, with a series of perspectives published in the *British Medical Journal*, supporting community initiatives, specialist services, primary health-care work, and the need for a research base (Bewley 1967; Connell 1967; Chapple 1967; Owens 1967). There was general agreement on the need for treatment to be available in the community. As Owens said, 'narcotic addiction must be regarded primarily as a problem of community mental health' (Owens 1967). Indeed the whole focus of the *British Medical Journal* contribution from Chapple was on treatment in the community (Chapple 1967). However, as both Connell and Bewley pointed out (Bewley 1967; Connell 1967) there was a reluctance on the part of medical colleagues to be involved in provision of treatment and hence there was a strong argument for the establishment of special centres, which should be located in areas with established addiction problems, and based in teaching hospitals with back-up laboratory and in-patient facilities. Indeed, treatment should extend beyond these centres so that experimental hostels might be set up 'to provide support and supervision for the addict, and gradually to introduce him to and integrate him into the community and to prevent him going back to the addict sub-culture' (Connell 1967).

Addict voices appeared for the first time in the popular press (*Sunday Times* 1966; Trocchi 1965); public interest was considerable and included concern at the excessive prescribing by a small number of doctors, to such an extent that television was the new medium for the cross-examination and 'trial' by David Frost of prescribing doctors such as Dr John Petro (described in Judson 1974).

The new response

Through 1967 the Ministry of Health was preparing plans for the creation of the new treatment centres. As Stimson and Oppenheimer (1982) were subsequently to comment, the new clinics were required to walk a prescribing tightrope, with the dangers of overprescribing (and hence feeding the black market) on the one hand, and the danger of under-prescribing (and hence failing to capture and contain the problem) on the other side. The blueprint for the new clinics was contained within the memorandum from the Ministry of Health (1967) entitled 'Treatment and supervision of heroin addiction', in which there was a recognition of the need to achieve this balance on the prescribing tightrope. The aim of the new clinics was 'to contain the spread of heroin addiction by continuing to supply the drug in minimum quantities where this is necessary in the opinion of the doctor, and where possible to persuade addicts to accept withdrawal treatment' (Ministry of Health 1967). Edwards (1969) later described how clinicians aimed to 'with one hand give the addict heroin, while with the other hand build his motivation to come off the drug'. There was a determination to see the new clinics as providing something much more than just hand-outs of drugs. A *Lancet* editorial (1968) conveyed the strong determination that the clinics should be adequately staffed so as to be able to practise an energetic and comprehensive approach – not just the dispensing of drugs. In similar vein, Edwards outlined how vitally important it would be that staff of the new clinics

> should be concerned with and involved in the total treatment programme, should have as their aim to woo the addict off drugs, and must have immediately available facilities for detoxification and later rehabilitation, so that, when the addict shows interest in treatment, treatment can be provided. The doctors staffing these clinics cannot be part-time clinical assistants unsupported by psychiatric training.
>
> (Edwards 1967)

The rationale of the new approach

In an account written in the months leading up to the opening of the new treatment clinics, Connell (1969) summarized the rationale of the new approach as follows:

> (i) the addict is a sick person and properly comes within the ambit of medical practice: his dependence on the drug and his craving are so strong that he is unable to behave rationally;
> (ii) heroin will be provided free at special treatment centres: this will obviate the necessity for acquisitive crime to pay for the drug from the blackmarket which was not yet criminally well organised;
> (iii) NHS staff in the new treatment centres will be less likely to over-prescribe, and will use the opportunity of contact with the addict to cultivate motivation towards eventual withdrawal from the drug: regular contact between the addict and the doctor of the treatment clinic will provide the opportunity for a relationship to be built-up which may eventually lead to the addict requesting to be taken off the drug;
> (iv) the prescribing of heroin by the treatment centres should so under-cut the blackmarket as to prevent its development or consolidation;
> (v) a more careful approach will be taken to matching dose pre-scribed to dose needed so that there would be much less 'spare' heroin circulating to involve less committed individuals;

(vi) punitive detention of the addict under a penal system has not been shown to be successful in curing addiction in other countries.

(Connell 1969)

Thus it was intended that a safe middle path would be trod between the two extremes of prescribing, so as to achieve adequate impact at the levels of both individual care and social control.

In a later commentary on the new clinics, Edwards (1969) put forward three hypotheses relating to the treatment being provided:

(i) Addicts are taken on by the clinics not for the continuing handouts of drugs, but for treatment: the patient may not initially be motivated to accept withdrawal but, through contact with clinic staff, motivation will gradually be built, dosage gradually reduced, and the offer of admission for withdrawal finally accepted.

(ii) Since successful treatment ultimately depends on the patient's own motivation, there is no place for the use of compulsory admission procedures.

(iii) There are believed to be some patients who cannot – or cannot for the time being – function without the drug, but who on a regular maintenance dose can live a normal and useful life as a 'stabilized addict': such patients will be maintained on heroin rather than have their drug withdrawn.

(Edwards 1969)

One further recommendation had been put forward in the Second Report from the Brain Committee – the only recommendation not to be implemented. It had been proposed that doctors should be given the power to detain addicts compulsorily in hospital (under, for example, a new provision of the Mental Health Act). However, despite attracting occasional support (for example, Bewley 1967), other more sceptical voices prevailed (for example, Connell 1967; *Lancet* 1968) and no such powers were agreed, for fear that too hasty provision of such compulsory powers might lead to widespread use of these powers which were not necessary or were likely to be ineffective or even counter-productive.

The new services

Fifteen out-patient clinics were opened across London, most of them attached to teaching hospitals. Additionally, a smaller number of clinics were opened in towns near to London. Very few specialist clinics were set up elsewhere in the UK. Some of these new clinics were open every weekday whilst others were only open part-time. Almost overnight, working policies and practices needed to be developed. During the first year of operation regular meetings were arranged by the Ministry of Health for the doctors in charge of the new treatment centres across the country. Accounts of the practice of individual clinics were published at the time (for example, Gardner and Connell 1970) and a contemporary account summarizing the first year was later published (Connell 1991). A degree of control was introduced – for example, addicts now had to attend weekly or fortnightly out-patient appointments and were usually required to collect their drugs on a daily basis from a local pharmacist. Such developments were viewed by many addicts as 'an absolute bore' (quote from Christina Boyd, interviewed by Stimson and Oppenheimer 1982), even though the degree of individual freedom, with take-home supplies, injectable drugs, and fixing rooms and free equipment in several of the clinics was still a world apart from the more controlled treatment approaches of most other countries.

The dangers of the new approach

From the very outset it was recognized that considerable navigational skill would be required in negotiating a safe passage between the dangers of over-control and under-control which lay on either side. Concerns were voiced – for example, in the *British Medical Journal*: 'One has fears for treatment centres – for example, one dreads that they will merely become prescribing centres . . .' (Owens 1967). Contemporary accounts (Connell 1969; Edwards 1969) are clear illustrations of the awareness of the brinkmanship in which they were engaged. It was necessary to identify and face these dangers in order to 'avoid a drift into disaster and a breakdown of the new approach' (Connell 1969). Amongst others, the following weak points in the system were identified by Connell (1969):

(i) It had already been demonstrated that a very small number of over-prescribing doctors could encourage an epidemic of drug taking when it coincided with a socio-cultural demand.
(ii) The new 'experts' did not have tools for precise measurement of the dose required for each patient.
(iii) All professional classes contain weaker brethren.
(iv) The new planned response had required the recruitment of many more doctors into the practice of prescribing heroin to addicts.

(Connell 1969)

These conflicts were graphically illustrated at the time by various commentaries. For example, Edwards (1969) cited two cases to illustrate the difficulties facing the prescriber:

A 17 year old girl who was on 30 mg of heroin and 40 mg of methadone per day was in physiological balance but insisted that she wanted a bigger prescription: an increased dose was refused, so she went to the blackmarket and built her dose up to 120 mg of heroin per day, as was confirmed when she was admitted for stabilisation. Because her story had not been believed, she had meanwhile certainly been receiving an insufficient script for maintenance and had been driven into criminal activities in a way which the legalised prescribing system is supposed to circumvent. The second case was an addict on 90 mg of heroin per day who complained bitterly on Monday of the clinic's callous under-prescribing which, she stated, was making any sort of social adjustment impossible; later the same week, she was arrested for selling the drug.

(Edwards 1969)

The development of safeguards

In his contemporary analysis, Connell (1969) identified two main strategies for cutting down the pool of surplus heroin which might influence the uninitiated or uncommitted heroin user. First, it was proposed that doses of drugs already being prescribed to addicts should be reduced gradually down to more moderate levels (daily doses for some addicts had climbed astronomically – to doses many times greater than the maximum doses found necessary in other more experienced countries). By this approach, the absolute quantity of drug involved in any small diversions of supplies would represent fewer unit doses for the novice or uncommitted user. Second, the practice of clinics should be such as to promote downward rather than upward changes to the dose prescribed. Previous independent doctors had been caught in a spiralling increase of dose as tolerance developed. The downward perspective involved a recognition that addicts have two needs: a physiological need to prevent withdrawal symptoms and a psychological need to obtain the 'high' associated with increased dose: the former should be adequately addressed by stable or even slowly reducing dose, whereas attempts to satisfy the latter need would lead to continuing dose escalation. Gradually an informal code of practice was established (for the 1969 contemporary account which was later published see Connell 1991), although this was not a static code of practice but represented the consensus or prevailing view based on practice and experience as it was accrued. In the early 1980s, when interest in the provision of care to opiate addicts again became a subject of public and medical interest, a later code of practice was published from the London clinics (Connell and Mitcheson 1984) and was followed shortly afterwards by Guidelines of good clinical practice from the Department of Health (Medical Working Group on Drug Dependence 1984).

This 1969 informal code of practice included recommendations for weekly or fortnightly interview/assessment of the patient; the posting of prescriptions to a local community pharmacist by prior arrangement; the dispensing of a day's supply of drugs at a time by this community pharmacist; the dispersal of addicts over as large a number of chemists as practical so as to prevent the congregation of addicts at key pharmacies. Once the dust had settled from the transfer of care of the established addicts who had been in receipt of private prescriptions, a more cautious approach was adopted for assessment of the new patient prior to the commencing of prescribing heroin or cocaine – and indeed cases were identified in which the initial enthusiasm (on the part of the prescriber as well as the patient) for commencement of the prescription had led to the prescribing of opiates to non-addicted individuals (Gardner and Connell 1970).

During the first year of operation many of the doctors in charge of the treatment centres formed the view that the continued prescribing of injectable cocaine was unnecessary due to the absence of a recognized withdrawal syndrome. When addicts presented in an emergency in opiate withdrawal, the withdrawal syndrome should be managed with linctus methadone in a dose sufficient to cover the patient until his next appointment – a policy adopted partly in order to prevent the development of such emergency presentations as a loophole for obtaining extra supplies of heroin. Agreement was also reached between the treatment centres about consultation before transfer of patients between clinics so as to prevent patients from 'shopping around' solely to obtain the highest offer of a prescribed dose.

During their first few months, the clinics took over the care of all the heroin addicts who had been obtaining their supplies from the private and National Health Service GPs. From 16 April 1968 onwards, supplies of heroin or cocaine to addicts were all channelled through the new treatment centres. It seems likely that during the transition period there was considerable overprescribing, in that most patients were taken on with a dose of drugs similar to their previous care. Gradually, individual cases and individual dose requirement could be assessed by the clinics so as to identify grosser abuses of the system. Even during the first 18 months, one particular clinic had experienced something of a local epidemic which appeared to stem from internal traffic of patients within the clinic system towards the more liberal prescribing policy of this clinic.

For a while, an additional problem occurred with the prescribing of injectable amphetamine. By mid-1968, once the new clinics had taken over care of the heroin addicts, two private doctors began 'prescribing quantities of the drug (methylamphetamine ampoules) to an extent which contributed directly to the growth of the illicit market' (Hawks et al. 1969). A brief experiment of prescribing supplies of methylamphetamine ampoules seemed to be 'largely a record of therapeutic failure' (Mitcheson et al. 1976), and by the end of 1968 agreement was reached between the Department of Health and the pharmaceutical manufacturers so that the drug was withdrawn from supply to retail chemists. This intervention would appear to have been highly effective and successfully aborted the growing intravenous amphetamine problem (for analysis, see de Alarcon 1972).

At the end of this interim period, it was evident that both addicts and the clinics had survived the transition period, but there remained fundamental issues which still needed to be addressed (contemporary data collected in 1969 – later published in Connell 1991). To what extent should the clinics look for more evidence of use and dependence prior to commencing a prescription? What approach should be adopted to the new methadone ampoules (for which a special licence to prescribe was not required)? What policy should be adopted for the increasing number of primary methadone addicts (those who have never taken heroin before their methadone use)? And what should be the policy with those individuals dependent on other drugs (such as amphetamines, barbiturates, etc.) or with non-injecting drug addicts – should they be treated within the same service, in parallel services or in separate services?

The challenge

The new drug problem in the 1960s undoubtedly represented a major challenge to the formerly quiet British System. What was the nature of the challenge faced by the new clinics? In a paper written at the time of the opening of these new clinics, Connell (1969) identifies four particular challenges:

(1) the challenge to doctors in the new treatment centres to work together and adopt a reasonably uniform approach (and hence accept some restrictions on the practitioner's hallowed independence);
(2) the challenge to the biochemist to develop more rapid qualitative tests for drugs of abuse, and to develop methods for quantitative assessment of drug dosage;
(3) the challenge to medical practitioners to produce hard data relating to the different treatment programmes in order that effectiveness may be measured;
(4) the challenge to epidemiologists and sociologists to produce data relating to the causes, method of spread, and options for prevention of drug taking.

(Connell 1969)

Conclusions

Without doubt, the opening of the clinics on 16 April 1968 was a major point of change in the relationship between the addict and the doctor in the UK. Addicts themselves had changed rapidly (in epidemiological terms) from the middle-aged addicts of the previous decades (predominently therapeutic addicts and health-care professionals) to the new young addicts born of the 1960s revolution. The change in the treatment response was a result of revision of policy over a similar time-span of a few years, and was implemented virtually overnight. As Bill Gregor said (addict patient interviewed by Stimson and Oppenheimer, 1982): 'When the clinics started, the heyday, if you can call it that, was over'. Certainly the scope for the more excessive abuses of the British freedom to prescribe had been curbed, but what was the nature of the altered British System which grew in the new climate? Within a health-care context, a complicated script had been written for the new clinics which involved simultaneous concern about broader social and public health perspectives on the one hand and treatment of the individual patient on the other. The struggle to reconcile these two seemingly contradictory goals formed the basis of work and evolution of the British clinics during the next decade (see Stimson and Oppenheimer 1982; and Chapters 3 and 4, this volume), and the debate about the balance between these two goals has re-emerged during the late 1980s and early 1990s with the new analysis required in the wake of HIV/AIDS (see Advisory Council on the Misuse of Drugs 1988, 1989; Strang and Stimson 1990; Power *et al.* 1991; see also Chapters 11 and 16 in Volume I). Much of the rhetoric, policy consideration and clinical practice of today is strongly reminiscent of the events around the time of the creation of the clinics – and yet, sadly, scant regard is paid to perspectives from yester-year. Perhaps the ignorant must be condemned to repeat the agonies, the considerations, and the errors of history without reference to previous journeys through similarly turbulent waters.

References

Advisory Council on the Misuse of Drugs (1988). AIDS and drug misuse. Part 1. HMSO, London.

Advisory Council on the Misuse of Drugs (1989). AIDS and drug misuse. Part 2. HMSO, London.

Bewley, T. (1967). Centres for the treatment of addiction: advantages of special centres. *British Medical Journal*, 2, 498–99.

Chapple, P. A. L. (1967). Centres for the treatment of addiction: treatment in the community. *British Medical Journal*, 2, 500–1.

Connell, P. H. (1967). Centres for the treatment of addiction: importance of research. *British Medical Journal*, 2, 499–500.

Connell, P. H. (1969). Drug dependence in Great Britain: a challenge to the practice of medicine. In *Scientific basis of drug dependence* (ed. H. Steinberg). Churchill Livingstone, London.

Connell, P. H. (1991). Treatment of drug-dependent patients 1968–1969 (Document). *British Journal of Addiction*, 86, 913–16.

Connell, P. H. and Mitcheson, M. (1984). Necessary safeguards when prescribing opioid drugs to addicts: experience of drug dependence clinics in London. *British Medical Journal*, 288, 767–9.

de Alarcon, R. (1969). The spread of heroin abuse in a community. *Bulletin on Narcotics*, 21, 17–22.

de Alarcon, R. (1972). An epidemiological evaluation of a public health measure aimed at reducing the availability of methylamphetamine. *Psychological Medicine*, 2, 293–300.

de Alarcon, R. and Rathod, N. H. (1968). Prevalence and early detection of heroin abuse. *British Medical Journal*, 1, 549–53.

Edwards, G. (1967). Relevance of American experience of narcotic addiction to the British scene. *British Medical Journal*, 3, 425–7.

Edwards, G. (1969). The British approach to the treatment of heroin addiction. *Lancet*, i, 768–72.

Frankau, I. M. and Stanwell, P. M. (1961). The treatment of heroin addiction. *Lancet*, ii, 1377–9.

Gardner, R. and Connell, P. H. (1970). One year's experience in a drug dependence clinic. *Lancet*, ii, 455–8.

Hawks, D. V., Mitcheson, M., Ogborne, A. and Edwards, G. (1969). Abuse of methylamphetamine. *British Medical Journal*, 2, 715–21.

Hewettson, J. and Ollendorf, R. (1964). Preliminary survey of 100 London heroin and cocaine addicts. *British Journal of Addiction*, 59, 109–14.

Interdepartmental Committee on Drug Addiction (The Brain Committee) (1961). Drug Addiction: report. HMSO, London.

Interdepartmental Committee on Drug Addiction (The Brain Committee) (1965). Drug Addiction: second report. HMSO, London.

Judson, H. (1974). *Heroin addiction in Britain*. Harcourt Brace Jovanovich, New York.

Kosviner, A., Mitcheson, M. C., Myers, K., Ogborne, A., Stimson, G. V., Zacune, J. and Edwards, G. (1968). Heroin use in a provincial town. *Lancet*, i, 1189–92.

Lancet (Editorial) (1968). Addiction new style. *Lancet*, i, 852–3.

Medical Working Group on Drug Dependence (1984). Guidelines of good clinical practice in the treatment of drug misuse. HMSO, London.

Ministry of Health (1967). Treatment and supervision of heroin addiction. Health Circular 67/16. Ministry of Health, London.

Mitcheson, M., Edwards, G., Hawks, D. and Ogborne, A. (1976). Treatment of methylamphetamine users during the 1968 epidemic. In *Drugs and drug dependence* (eds G. Edwards, M. Russell, D. Hawks and M. McCafferty), pp. 155–62. Saxon House/Lexington, Farnborough.

Owens, J. (1967). Centres for treatment of drug addiction: integrated approach. *British Medical Journal*, 2, 501–2.

Power, R., Stimson, G. V. and Strang, J. (1991). Drug prevention and HIV policy. *AIDS* 1990, 4 (suppl. 1), S263–7.

Rolleston Committee (Departmental Committee on Morphine and Heroin Addiction) (1926). Report. HMSO, London.

Spear, H. B. (1969). The growth of heroin addiction in the United Kingdom. *British Journal of Addiction*, 64, 245.

Stimson, G. V. and Oppenheimer, E. (1982). *Heroin addiction: treatment and control in Britain*. Tavistock, London.

Strang, J. and Stimson, G. V. (1990). The impacts of HIV: forcing the process of change. In *AIDS and drug misuse: the challenge for policy and practice in the 1990s* (ed. J. Strang and G. V. Stimson), pp. 3–15. Routledge, London.

Sunday Times (1966). Heroin addiction. *Sunday Times*, 6 March.

Trocchi, A. (1965). Why drugs? *New Society*, 5 (138), 1–2.

Zacune, J. (1971). A comparison of Canadian narcotic addicts in Great Britain and Canada. *Bulletin on Narcotics*, 23, 41–9.

Chapter 3

The new drug clinics of 1968

'Everything will be alright when the new place is built'

James Willis

Preamble

This is a personal memoir of the early days of the St Giles' Drug Dependence Unit (DDU) which opened in south London in 1967. I was its Director until 1976 when I left the NHS to work overseas. The clinic was one of the DDUs set up when the law was changed, limiting the prescribing of diamorphine and cocaine in the treatment of addiction, to physicians licensed by the Home Office.

Introduction

When the proposed legal changes had been agreed, the first response was to set up clinics in the London area. Each clinic would be linked to a teaching hospital. It was hoped that this would provide a solid base for the clinics, readier access to staffing and funding, and a basis for data collection which would contribute to a better understanding of the nature and extent of the problem. The clinics would be under the direction of a consultant psychiatrist, and staffed by a multi-disciplinary team. So far, so good. What no one had reckoned with was that the clinics might not be welcomed by certain psychiatrists who had the (unfounded) suspicion that they might be told what to do by unspecified administrators. This resistance immediately suggested to me that the whole enterprise was likely to be shaky from the start, since some of the psychiatrists involved were concerned that they might be corralled into a style of practice that was not to their liking and flounce off in a huff. Or if they didn't feel that way, their psychiatric colleagues, outside the field of drug dependence, were sometimes only too ready to suggest that this was how it might go.

Also, even over thirty years later, it is hard to convey the amount of concern that the 'Drug Menace' had engendered. From day one the psychiatrists in the DDUs were to be watched by the media, by social scientists and criminologists, by the clergy; by an army of the well-meaning, and most of all by their colleagues. It seemed as if everyone was waiting for us to screwup. However, despite daily criticism of our failure to solve the problem, sweep it under the carpet, or whatever we were expected to do, I believe that our people did their best to set up programmes which evolved gradually and changed radically in the process. It was a brave attempt to tackle a little understood problem, by a group of well-intentioned persons who were not motivated by personal gain beyond their NHS salaries. Furthermore, it was not, as has sometimes been represented, an attempt to railroad patients into a coercive system with no regard for anything beyond arguments over prescriptions. A general impression has been created that the system was 'uncaring'. Those who have suggested this have done a disservice to the people concerned. It wasn't like that at all. Caring for patients isn't all about touchy-feeliness and emotional incontinence.

My personal experience

In 1966, I was a consultant at Warlingham Park Hospital. Amongst others, I was asked for my opinion about the proposed clinics, and also whether I would be interested in applying for a post in one. I was dubious about the idea. My interest in drug dependence was a sideline which had become a welcome diversion from a certain ennui that was spreading through mental hospital consultant life; fear of dissolution, bickering committees and pointless discussions about whether nurses ought to wear uniform or ordinary clothing. My entry on the scene was almost accidental. In 1964 I had started interviewing heroin users in London, and collecting data leading to the comparison of demographic features and the natural history of drug usage and criminality in London and New York addicts. I then started admitting addict patients to Stone House Hospital and later to Warlingham Park. In no time at all I became an 'expert'. Michael Shepherd told me I would be one in no time: I thought he was pulling my leg.

Appointment as consultant and the search for premises

One thing led to another, and I was appointed to the post of DDU consultant in 1967. I was told to get on with it. And I did. I thought the first thing to do was take over patients from the independent prescribers, decent well-meaning guys who had done their best and got hammered by the media and many smug physicians. When Guy's had been approached, the late Dr David Stafford-Clark had come up with the idea of a joint clinic, with King's College Hospital providing an out-patient clinic and Bexley providing in-patient facilities. Guy's, in the event, offered the site for the out-patient clinic at St Olave's. A purpose-designed clinic was eventually built, but it was never occupied as the local population threatened to burn it down. This triumph for working-class fascism culminated in a public meeting chaired

by the then Minister of Health, with the local MP, Bob Mellish, in attendance. I was present on my own, with no representative from Guy's Hospital
available, until the late Lord Robens came along, of his own accord, to
provide me with the support that my own hospital apparently felt unable to
give. By then, in 1969, enthusiasm at the Guy's end was waning; the sight
of bedraggled addicts in the Psychiatric OPD had frightened the horses,
so to speak. And, to be fair, addicts did little to promote a positive public
image. Mr Mellish said that he could not guarantee that his constituents
would not attack the building, so I felt the best option was to let it go.
After the meeting, a rent-a-yob crowd stood at the gates of St Olave's, made
tribal noises and spat on my windscreen. I was also referred to as 'a Judas
in our midst' by the local press. It must have been the red hair, I suppose.
Happy days.

So, after this unhappy setback, we returned to a search for 'temporary
premises'. These included a variety of run-down premises, the Red Cross
HQ in Peckham, and a disused building next door to the Bermondsey
Labour Party. It had been used as accommodation for building workers,
and had then become a squat from which the occupants had departed during
a nation-wide toilet-paper famine. The Labour Party soon put a block on
that one. Then, out of the blue, the St Giles' Centre offered King's College
Hospital the use of their premises. The Centre had been set up by the Revd
Chad Varah as a walk-in facility for meths drinkers from Camberwell Green,
but never got off the ground. It proved to be an instant fix and was rented
by KCH. This was preceded by a temporary stay in the Sexually Transmitted
Disease clinic unit at St Giles' Hospital. STD was a dead speciality in 1967.
It must seem hard to believe that nowadays. So was Infectious Disease, but
this was before immuno-compromised patients and HIV had proliferated.
Eventually we moved back to St Giles' Hospital, where the old STD clinic
had been converted into the St Giles' Clinic. So we stayed there. In retrospect,
I realise that we had a lucky escape when the St Olave's Clinic failed to
open. It would have been a disaster.

Getting it to work

Much has been said about the fact that there was no formal British System.
I think that this was a good thing. Suppose we had a British System, and
that it had been written down like the US constitution. If you look at the
dire effects this has had on many features of US society, there is a good
argument against a written constitution.

It was hard going at first, as I started on my own, and just took on the
patients and began a clean-up operation. This was a valuable lesson, since I
soon found out what a ghastly experience the prescribing general practitioners had endured, and that the management of addicts by the unsupported is
a hopeless task. At the in-patient end, everything went well from the start.

The looked-down-on-mental hospital, given no choice in the matter, came up trumps. Everyone at Bexley was generously open-handed to someone who had been foisted on them. Dr Ken Shaw allocated me Ashdown ward, and the nursing staff accepted me and my misfits without batting an eyelid. Dr Martin Mitcheson was great. He arrived on the doorstep at St Giles' in search of research material; saw how overloaded I was, and just got stuck in. I'll never forget his cheery support and real help. My spirits always rose when he poked his head round the door.

Patients – the population

An important problem, perhaps not clearly enough appreciated by people in the field nowadays, is that, when the clinics were started, drug addiction had moved fairly rapidly from the status of a medical curiosity to a growing problem for which there was considerable public demand for relief, quite apart from medical and sociological concern. The available literature in this country was sparse and anecdotal, and the American literature, though expanding, had not reached the level of sophistication and scientific credibility that is found today. The epidemiology of the problem in the 1960s was in the process of being mapped out, and remained a source of speculation and controversy. The Home Office was criticised for understating the extent of the problem, the medical profession for indifference and tardiness; the air was thick with unverifiable assertions. And as usual, the voice of informed moderation was given little or no attention.

At first we had a large proportion of patients with major personality disorders; perhaps only to be expected at the beginning of an epidemic of severe risk-taking behaviour. Perhaps the first tobacco smokers were a similar population. I was struck by the change when in 1985 I returned to become Director of the Liverpool DDU and found the majority of our patients to be normal youngsters.

The patients we took on in the first days of the clinics were, on the whole, in very bad shape. Patients with arms and legs covered in needle tracks, dirty, unkempt and lice-ridden were the norm. There was a general idea, fostered by the media, that many bogus addicts would be taken on and given drugs that they did not need, so that they could sell them. My experience was that such phonies were infrequent, and easily spotted, including one reporter from a national daily newspaper. It may be imagined that the early days were edgy and uncertain. On the one hand we had a patient population that was apprehensive, and often angry; on the other hand, a group of wary and inexperienced physicians; on the sidelines was an interested public, amongst whom real concern competed with prurience. Some atmosphere in which to start a new service, one might think.

The first patients to be taken on at St Giles' were handed over by doctors who had known their patients reasonably well, and they were able to give me reliable indications as to who could be trusted and who not. This meant taking on a large number of patients relatively abruptly, but I felt that it was best to make the transfer, let the dust settle, and then establish a reliable records system. Patients were told that their prescriptions would be left as they were at entry until further decisions could be made, when I had got to know them better. This worked out well in that the majority of the patients taken on were 'old-timers' who slotted into the system fairly easily. On the appointed day, the doctors met me at the STD clinic at St Giles', introduced me to the remaining patients on their list of addicts, handed me their prescription pads, and that was that.

The most difficult problems arose from patients who had been street junkies under the 'care' of Dr Petro, and those who had been buying heroin from them. They were an unknown quantity. The policy was to take them on probation, and see how things worked out. In this way it proved possible to weed out those who were selling half or more of the drugs prescribed. As might be imagined, this was often a stormy process, especially at first when I was on my own, and seemingly inundated. But this position improved as soon as staffing was established in the first six months.

Certain patients had found my home telephone number, and in the first weeks the phone seemed to ring all night about 'lost' drugs, etc., but a few stern warnings put a stop to it. The police at West End Central would ring during the night about patients stopped and searched in W1, and found to be in possession, etc. My wife had some interesting comments when a PC would call at three in the morning and ask if she were my secretary. Those early days were fairly awful, but I was enthusiastic, as we all were. This point is worth stressing. I believe that we all entered the system full of high hopes.

General medical services

General practitioners were understandably wary of addicts, and so we provided general medical care. Hospital admission, even for septicaemia, was sometimes difficult to arrange, as hospitals weren't keen on addicts on the wards. Also the patients were suspicious of hospitals. I was obliged to treat patients with septicaemia as out-patients. That was all I could do. Nowadays disruptive behaviour by addicts and drunks is commonplace in A&E departments, but the amphetamine-high junkie storming around demanding drugs was a new and alarming experience, as insoluble today as then. It is merely that it is now part of the scenery. Eventually, the real heroes were the junior physicians and nurses in local hospitals who took a chance and admitted patients, also certain consultants who were prepared to have a go. Physicians and surgeons were often far more tolerant than psychiatrists. In general the worst physicians, as far as their reaction to addicts were concerned, were a few psychiatrists who remained lofty and judgemental towards the patients and towards the 'Drug Doctors', who represented the dirty end of psychiatry as far as they were concerned.

This provided tasty fodder for the social scientists.

Staffing

On one occasion, at the Royal College of Physicians, I had been asked to give a talk about the work of a Drug Addiction Unit, and started off with the words 'I am a Drug Addiction Unit.' At that stage it was true. I was holding three clinics a week in the old STD clinic at St Giles' on my own, except for visits from a kindly woman from medical records who tried to arrange an appointments system. She took up the cause, as she'd been led to believe that the clinic would be a scene of God knows what varieties of orgiastic behaviour. She found that it was mainly populated by those in deep faeces, and spread the word that it wasn't as bad as all that, and that I was a decent chap. This helped. The next person to come along was Peter the porter. He was assigned to me to act as a minder. He was an amazing find, as it turned out. Nothing fazed him. He had an air of quiet authority and could calm potential aggression by poking his head around the door and saying, 'Everything all right, Dr Willis?' He was a Para in the Territorial RAMC. He was also an excellent information source and soon got to know who was dealing, etc. Another of his self-appointed tasks was to get people to tidy themselves up. 'Go and get a shave,' he'd say. 'Dr Willis is in there in a nice suit so why don't you go and clean yourself up a bit. If he goes to that trouble, so can you. Show respect.' Thus I became a role model; raising fears that I might be showered with stolen cuff-links at Christmas.

Three Clinical Assistants were appointed, two at St Giles' and one at Bexley. Again I was very lucky in that they were mature, experienced doctors who were able, *inter alia*, to provide general medical services to the patients. This is an important point to mention, as it was difficult for addicts to receive medical care. Many were vagrants, living in squats and giving false names and non-existent addresses. Then we acquired a Research Fellow/Medical Assistant who switched to SHMO grade. She was MD PhD, and hitherto had been in gastro-enterology. At the same time we took on board two social workers, both American, with some experience of drug-related problems. There is no doubt that at first social workers found the clinics more daunting than did the medical staff. This is hardly surprising, given the prevailing philosophy of social work at that time. My attitude was that, in view of our general lack of experience, social workers should be given an open cheque book and allowed to get on with things.

One of the most fortuitous appointments was a secretary who was appointed in 1970 and stayed with the clinic after it closed and changed to a community-based service. Margot Benady was a key person at the clinic. She was the ideal person to be the first point of contact for anyone, be they patients or visiting big shots, towards whom she displayed calm impartiality. She had a special qualification – perfect manners.

In the early days the whole operation was clinic-based and there was no community involvement. This was obviously far from satisfactory, but it was a start at a time when there was clamour for quick solutions. It took time for people to accept the notion that these services can only be developed gradually. I saw our role as one of triage and first aid, until we got to know the patient population. An unexpected feature of clinic life in the early days was the constant stream of visitors, many from the United States, including criminologists, lawyers and police. Medical students came on elective appointments. I found this a good experience, since I was soon forced to answer questions about what we were doing. It was often hard for me to give satisfactory answers, since none of us, at that stage, had a clear idea how things would turn out. Were we wasting our time in maintenance programmes? Should we switch from heroin maintenance to methadone? Why were we not being more aggressive in our search for abstinence? Being put up against the ropes with such questions, I was obliged to examine what we were doing.

Data collection and investigations

The patients taken on at the start were an unknown population, so the first task was to piece together proper histories, and assess physical and mental status. This involved simple history taking, and the use of standard data-recording protocols. Other agencies became involved. The Liver Unit from KCH started a prospective study of hepatic function and hepatitis B prevalence. Needle-transmitted jaundice was prevalent; its extent required exploration. We had visits from a dermatologist interested in the skin infections, abscesses, etc., that were commonplace, as were ulcers caused by the injection of crushed-up barbiturate tablets. Workers from the Addiction Research Unit at the Institute of Psychiatry included our patient population in their surveys, so that by the end of the first three years it could be said that our 250-odd patients had become one of the most intensively researched groups around. In addition, one of our physicians made detailed studies of the physical status of the patients and found that, leaving aside their bedraggled appearance, they were a surprisingly healthy group. At the end of seven years we were able to produce a modest outcome study. Of the 250 original patients, seven had died, and the incidence of septicaemia and needle-borne infections, jaundice, etc. had fallen dramatically. Fifteen per cent had quit drug usage. And in general, drug usage had been reduced and the patient population was less panicky and explosive. We had all chilled out.

Special drug-related problems

Amphetamines

At first the amphetamines were our worst problem, in that most patients were receiving regular scripts for injectable methylamphetamine (methedrine). The associated behavioural disturbance, and the slipping in and out of psychosis, made it obvious that this was a practice that had to be stopped. As soon as it stopped, the clinics and the street drug scene calmed down within days. Ours did. Abusive behaviour, mainly verbal, was a constant problem, though actual physical assault occurred on only a few occasions. But until methylamphetamine was removed from the scene there was a constant air of menace that hung around many patients in states of chronic paranoid tension.

Methadone

All the clinics started prescribing methadone from the beginning, both as a medication to cover withdrawal and as a maintenance drug. At first, methadone seemed to be the pharmacological answer to many of the problems of heroin dependence. I had the opportunity of visiting the first methadone programme in New York and, like everyone else, had been most impressed by its dramatic effects in long-term users who had been stabilised, were working and had re-settled into a normal non-drug-using way of life. As the clinics settled down there was a gradual move towards replacing heroin with methadone. There is no doubt that all of us found methadone reduced heroin consumption, and helped the heroin user to lead a calmer, less disorganised life. I think that the main differences between clinics lay in the degree of insistence that we adopted towards the shift away from heroin to methadone. There was no general consensus on this for the first few years. And this may not have been a bad thing. We were all finding our way through uncharted territory.

At the same time there was a general rush to form confrontational therapeutic communities on the Phoenix House model. In truth I believe we were ready to try anything, and that in doing so we frequently bought ourselves a poor deal, especially in the days when it seemed that anyone from America had to know the answers, and that in the process, psychopathy was occasionally mistaken for charisma, as the grotesque absurdities of certain confrontational therapies revealed themselves. The Emperor's new clothes are not confined to fable.

Cocaine

We only had two long-term cocaine users. Both were Americans with histories going back over twenty and forty years respectively. They are now both dead. One died in her late sixties of lung cancer, and the other died of end-stage renal failure. He had refused dialysis. He was an aggressive psychopath who claimed to have been in a chain gang in Georgia, in his time. There were times when I wished he had stayed there. All other patients on cocaine were taken off straight away.

Hypno-sedatives

The barbiturates, especially the quinalbarbitone/amylobarbitone hybrid 'Tuinal' and the non-barbiturate sedative, methaqualone, caused many severe problems when they were prescribed by a series of rogue doctors, an interesting group of miscreants and fools, out for a fast buck, who repeatedly fouled the nest. As soon as one disappeared, another would turn up and cause chaos before being snuffed out.

Rogue doctors

One of the most unusual of the rogue doctors of the 1960s was Dr X. I first heard about him from patients who had attended his clinic: e.g., 'I went up Dr X's din I?' He had suddenly acquired fame, later notoriety, because of his prescribing habits and the formation of a bogus anti-addiction society. He prescribed unlimited amounts of amphetamines to anyone who wanted them and appeared on TV making pious statements. Warning bells rang when a patient's parent described how the doctor had urinated in the wash basin in his surgery during an interview.

I attended a court hearing in Southend in which his prescribing had led to disaster and recognised him as a doctor whom I'd met briefly in 1964 when he was a registrar. He had been sent along to attend tutorials by his chief who had said, 'I don't know what to make of this guy; he seems to want to do everything at once. I suspect that he'll turn out to be a psychopath and we ought to get rid of him . . .' He turned out to be a smoothtalking young man, who looked and dressed like a car salesman. He was over-anxious to please and sought consultant status, planning to pass the MRCP, the DPM and undergo a training analysis, preferably in six months. I found him to be unteachable and wondered if he was hypomanic, and said so to his chief. But he disappeared abruptly the next week and that was that until he turned up as a rogue doctor. He finally ended up in Broadmoor.

Prescribing policies – how did they work and did they?

The clinics followed the mode of practice developed at All Saints Hospital in Birmingham by Dr John Owens. Prescriptions were not handled by patients but mailed to retail pharmacists where the patients collected their

medication. This practice has continued. It had advantages and disadvantages. I could never understand why no attempt was made to use hospital
pharmacy services, despite certain obvious drawbacks, unruly patients dis-
rupting busy out-patient pharmacies and so on. It was said that hospital
pharmacists resisted the idea.

'The end of the heyday of the addict life'

This was said shortly after the clinics started, and is true in the sense that
heroin was no longer available more or less for the asking. Once a system or
a programme is established, there have to be some ground rules, and there was
general agreement that we should try and exert rational control over prescribing heroin, in order not only to prevent spillage into a state-sponsored
black market, but also to avoid making addicts out of people who were not
severely dependent. Thus everyone had differing expectations. Some, but
not all, of the patients still hoped that they would be provided with heroin
more or less as a right, and a minority were abusive if refused, but they were
a minority. The Department of Health personnel hoped that it would relieve
them of a tiresome problem, and the Home Office were hopeful too. The
psychiatrists concerned had mixed expectations; we took the view that we
were dealing with patients with chronic and relapsing disorders and that one
should start by tidying patients up, taking proper histories, assessing their
physical status, etc. I know that I was regarded as having a *laissez-faire*
attitude, and can only say that I am a sceptic with little patience with zealots.

None of us was helped by the media, who predicted failure of the policy
and eagerly seized on the oracular pronouncements of the latest loony of the
month who had found a new cure for drug addiction. This point is worth
elaborating. At the day of the 'handover', the clinics overnight became the
focus of intense interest. The media, who had been denouncing 'over prescribing physicians', soon started asking for immediate solutions, and,
as might be expected, the clinics were criticised for prescribing, too much or
too little, not 'treating' the patients, but handing out drugs, etc. Certain
residents near the St Giles' Clinic timed the attendance of patients so that
the media were able to ask how we could hope to do anything if the patients
only spent a few minutes in the clinic, and so on. It proved useless to try and
explain that we were still at the stage of first-aid, so to speak. Everyone had
some criticism to offer, but the main thrust was that not enough was being
done to address deep-seated problems which underlay the addictive process.
This was ill-judged comment based on ignorance. From the first, the clinics
offered social work services, counselling, group therapy, indeed anything
they could lay their hands on. Certain clinics had to adopt a tougher line
than others because of their geographical location. I would challenge
anyone to tell me how they would have run the Charing Cross Clinic on a
'walk-in' basis in a hospital that was within walking distance of Piccadilly,

given the population of street addicts of that area. In general, it was agreed amongst us that we would try to reduce drug prescribing to the minimum compatible with avoidance of illicit drug use. And we all tried to do this in our different ways. In retrospect I believe that was a good thing. If we had all adhered to cast-iron schedules, I doubt if we would have learned, and in any case who was there to establish such schedules?

We had monthly meetings at the Department of Health. These were useful, but they seemed to develop into a competition to see who was prescribing the least heroin, and provided a platform for certain members to preach the word. But that didn't matter, for there was a great amount of goodwill and the feeling that we were all in it together, so to speak. We all felt that we were doing the best we could in trying circumstances.

Prescribing and policy

The first major advance was the withdrawal of methylamphetamine and the general agreement that prescribing cocaine was a non-starter. Within a few months it became apparent that the presence of amphetamine-intoxicated patients was impossible to contend with. Disruptive paranoid outbursts cannot be bought off with methedrine. If anything they get worse. So we agreed that from a given day we would discontinue the prescribing of injectable methedrine. This was a major advance. The clinics quietened down almost overnight. The numbers of cocaine users were small and this drug was withdrawn almost immediately, with a few exceptions being made for real long-term users. Fashions in drug use change amazingly quickly. Within two years, Bing Spear of the Home Office had assured me that you couldn't give cocaine away in the streets of London and he was probably right. Times change.

Bargaining and trust

A grey area. No addict is a good advertisement for the drug that he or she uses, to say the least. Smirnoff doesn't use photographs of chronic alcoholics to promote the sale of vodka, and any conscientious physician must feel misgivings about seeming to collude in a self-destructive process.

From the start, the physician had to develop a sense of clinical judgement in which there had inevitably to be a conflict between maintaining the health of the patient and keeping the patient straight, i.e. free from withdrawal symptoms and away from illicit drug usage. A task that is as good as impossible.

Most of us used a rule of thumb when deciding the amount of heroin to be prescribed; the assumption being that a person would overstate their needs by a factor of at least 30 per cent. I suspect 50 per cent might have been a better guess. The central problem that nags at the prescribing physician is that of colluding in self-destruction. An addict who becomes drug free is always in a much better state of health than when using drugs. This cannot be gainsaid. At its best, prescribing is making the best of a bad job. However, it is a way of helping the addict to buy time, a precious commodity.

Attrition

The Medical Model is not perfect but it has the merit of assuming that it is humane to regard drug dependence as an illness, even if it doesn't entirely meet the tightest definition of illness. It seems to me that it is acceptable to treat the condition as if it were an illness, so long as one doesn't get too carried away by the notion, and suppose that therefore it follows that only medical people can deal with it. The most useful feature of the medical model is that it enables one to see addiction as a chronic and relapsing disorder, and be on the lookout for ways of improving the patient's condition and chances of survival. In this way the management of addictive problems becomes an exercise in attrition, in which one tries always to seek out a spark of motivation for the patient to quit the addict life.

Needles and syringes

From the very start in 1967, St Giles' Clinic provided sterile disposable needles, syringes and water. I felt that this was the logical thing to do. If we were providing the drug, then we should see to it that the patient injected it dissolved in sterile water, as opposed to the water from the toilets in Piccadilly. I was severely criticised for this. If this was colluding in a destructive process, all I can say is that the incidence of infections fell away rapidly.

Typical days – 1967

At first the patients were mainly long-term users, fairly well stabilised on heroin. Within weeks an avalanche of new patients appeared from various agencies, the Home Office, voluntary organisations and new walk-in faces off the streets. The busiest clinic was on a Monday afternoon.

It started at 2 p.m. and often did not finish until 10 p.m. On one occasion Peter said, 'Do you know you saw seventy patients today?' However, it was possible to settle things down fairly quickly and operate a proper appointment system, once secretarial help arrived. The chaos of the first few months was gone.

By 1968 the clinic was running just like any other out-patient clinic except that the clientele was more demanding, more unpredictable and more bent on self-destruction than the average. But the panic was over and the clinic was more manageable.

Dr Thomas Bewley once said that our initial task was 'to bring back the boredom to addiction'. I think that this was a good point. A popular stereotype of the drug user had assigned a certain bogus glamour to the notion of a rebellious non-conformist, a member of 'the counter-culture' defiantly rejecting bourgeois norms, *et hoc genus omne*. Thomas Bewley's observation made sense when one was confronted by the miserable situation of the addicts, their low self-esteem and passive drift downwards.

Prescribing addictive drugs: legalising drugs?

Although it is beyond the remit of this chapter to go into detail on this topic, someone with coal-face experience ought to be permitted an opinion. Prescribing central stimulants such as cocaine and amphetamines just does not work: rapid increase in tolerance precludes stability. Maintenance prescribing of narcotics will never be easy, and although methadone had seemed to be about the best bet, we can no longer continue to ignore the sensible use of heroin as a maintenance drug. Put simply, heroin should never have been discarded. The reasons for dropping it were irrational and badly conceived, being related to an ill-considered notion of knowing what is best for the patient. The advocacy of legalisation and free availability of narcotics may seem unrealistic and simplistic, no matter what *The Economist* may say, but given the serial failures of the Drugs Wars, a radical approach to drug availability has to be given a fair trial. Economists are no better at predicting in their own field than are racing correspondents in theirs. But the notion cannot be shrugged aside, given the seemingly total failure of legal controls. At the same time, to date I haven't been aware of anyone who proposes deregulation of controlled drugs who has addressed the mind-boggling administrative problems that would ensue, quite apart from ruthless opposition from international drug marketeers.

Envoi

Dr Tooth, Principal Medical Officer in the Deparment of Health, wrote to me shortly after my appointment and, in wishing me well, expressed the hope that 'people of goodwill such as yourself will not become disillusioned . . .'. At the appointments committee, I was asked if I had any misgivings about spending the rest of my life prescribing heroin for addicts. I replied that it was unlikely that things would turn out like that, since I had never wanted to spend my professional life in one post.

In one of their best recordings Peter Cook asks Dudley Moore, 'What's the worst job you ever 'ad then?' To which Dud replies that it had to do with Jayne Mansfield and the disposal of lobsters. There were many occasions when I could have answered the question in one terse sentence. But those were on bad days. Nobody's perfect.

Chapter 4

Uncertainty within the drug clinics in the 1970s

Martin Mitcheson

(This chapter originally appeared in J. Strang and M. Gossop (eds) *Heroin Addiction and Drug Policy: The British System*, Oxford University Press, 1994.)

Specialist drug clinics came into being as a response to the numerically small, although in percentage terms startling, increase in the number of young adults injecting heroin during the 1960s. Their supply of heroin came from the diversion of heroin prescribed to established addicts by a small number of independent doctors (Brain Committee 1965). These doctors never numbered more than six in London and were mostly working in private practice. An unknown proportion of their patients sold some of their pre-scribed drugs on the 'grey market' thus initiating others into the habit. In the absence of other means of controlling the prescribing of these doctors, and the subsequent diversion of heroin, the prescribing of heroin and cocaine to addicts was restricted to specially licensed doctors who worked at the new clinics which had been instituted at selected hospitals, mostly in London and including one private clinic. Effectively they became the only source in the UK of a heroin prescription for an addict.

The early days

The staff at the clinics had varied experience in working with drug misusers. Some had no previous experience. Regular meetings of the doctors in charge of clinics were instituted for sharing information and agreeing informal policies on such matters as appropriate assessment or what procedures should regulate the transfer of patients from one clinic to another (Connell 1991). Statistical information was provided at these meetings, regarding the number of patients receiving prescriptions at each clinic and the total quantity of heroin and methadone prescribed from each clinic. Even prior to the advent of cheap pocket calculators it was relatively easy for doctors attending these meetings to calculate a mean dose of opioids per patient for each clinic (see

Figures 4.1, 4.2 and 4.3). Given the overt reason for the establishment of clinics, which was to restrict the diversion of heroin to the grey market while allowing a sufficient continued 'ration' to established addicts, it was possible to see these meetings as typically English, discreet peer group pressure tending to moderate the prescribing of heroin. The alternative drug considered more acceptable by clinic staff was methadone – a longer acting synthetic opiate – which had a respectable image resulting from Dole *et al.* (1966) and their advocacy of methadone for maintenance in New York City. However, London addicts were accustomed to collecting supplies of injectable drugs from a retail pharmacy for self-injecting in private and they expected this practice to continue. Thus ampoules of methadone (Physeptone, 'Phy') injection were requested and prescribed. These were used in a manner very different from the USA, where clinics supervised consumption of oral methadone on the premises.

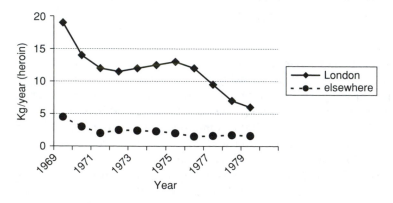

Figure 4.1 Bulk quantities of heroin prescribed annually: London alone; and rest of England
Source: Previously unpublished data supplied by the London Consultants Group.

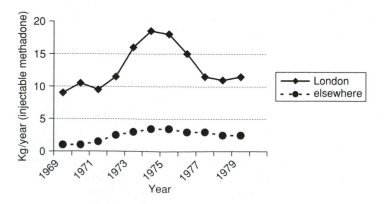

Figure 4.2 Bulk quantities of injectable methadone prescribed annually: London alone; and rest of England
Source: As Figure 4.1.

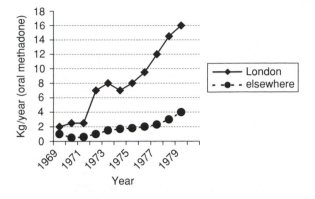

Figure 4.3 Bulk quantities of oral methadone prescribed annually: London alone; and rest of England
Source: As Figure 4.1.

Client contact and expectations

The early months of the clinics saw a rush of customers, who, correctly, anticipated that the initial launch of the clinics presented an opening offer to sign up for a maintenance prescription that might not be repeated. At the same time members of the street subculture rightly suspected that amounts prescribed by salaried clinic staff might be less generous than the prescriptions of independent practitioners. On the day in April 1968 that the new restrictive regulations came into force, *The Times* carried a report from a self-styled addiction specialist, with dubious qualifications, that the grey market price of diverted heroin had doubled from £1 to £2 for a grain of heroin (approximately 64 mg). Heroin was dispensed as one-sixth of a grain (approximately 10 mg) hypodermic tablets for injection. (These were subsequently replaced by freeze-dried ampoules in the late 1970s.) Expressed as pence per milligram, the price of diverted heroin increased from 1.5 p/mg, at which it had been traded between heroin users over the previous decade, to 3 p/mg.

From 1968, many clinics substituted ampoules of methadone for injection (supplied under the trade name Physeptone) instead of the heroin previously prescribed by independent doctors. It was not initially attempted to substitute oral methadone, as would then have been normal practice in the United States.

Initial customer reaction to 'Phy. amps' (ampoules of injectable methadone) was that they were only good for rinsing out one's 'works'. This rapidly gave way to a general realization that intravenous methadone was a rapid acting drug with euphoriant properties and the price of 10 mg units of injectable heroin and methadone rapidly achieved parity.

Staffing of the clinics

The clinics were sparsely staffed with part-time doctors, with varying supporting staff, including nurses, perhaps a social worker and receptionist/
secretarial support. Psychologists worked part-time in two London clinics
during this period. The clients' initial perceptions of clinics were principally
as a legitimate controlled source of drugs – and a cynical comment on the
parsimonious staffing would be that perhaps this view was shared by the
funding authorities. However, the staff, being mainly doctors and nurses,
strove to offer a more curative regimen. They offered, where possible: in-
patient as well as out-patient detoxification (although one London health
region then had no designated in-patient specialist drug unit and, indeed, in
1992 still had none); medical care; counselling; and social support, in several
cases developing specific links with non-statutory 'street agencies' as a form
of outreach foreshadowing the later development of Community Drug Teams.
Nevertheless an inordinate and wearisome amount of time was spent in
(usually polite) mutual manipulation between staff and patients regarding
type of drug and dose. Many clinics provided a room where patients could
inject the prescribed drugs with a degree of care, rather than lock themselves
in the lavatory to inject (Stimson 1973).

Questioning the therapeutic goal

By 1970 it was apparent to many clinic staff that for the majority of out-
patients attending clinics their physical health and social functioning was
not converted, by the receipt of a legitimate supply of heroin, to the behaviour
exhibited by the traditional middle-class therapeutic addict who had been
the mainstay of the traditional British System (Schur 1963).

It should be noted that Schur's description of the British System to which
he attributed the relatively low level of criminal activity by English drug
users was based on his experience in the late 1950s when he undertook his
research during a period at the London School of Economics. At that time
young heroin users were rare compared with the older patient wholly addicted to other opiates in the course of medical treatment. He did, however,
comment that in north London there was already a subcultural use of heroin,
with associated drug argot, which was more akin to the American experience
and had the potential for developing a different style of drug use. A contrary
view to that of Schur who advocated the 'British System' as maintaining a
low level of criminality was that presented by Larrimore and Brill (1967).
They made several visits to the UK, and suggested that it was the bourgeois
middle class, and previous non-criminal character of the traditional British
prescribed addict, which enabled the 'British System' to distribute legitimate
injectable heroin on medical prescription without the development of a social
drug problem.

Questioning the prescribing of injectable drugs

To examine the consequences over one year of a prescription of injectable heroin by comparison with a refusal to prescribe injectable drugs while offering oral methadone maintenance, a random controlled study was undertaken by this author at University College Hospital – the subjects being followed independently in the community by Richard Hartnoll (Mitcheson and Hartnoll 1978; Hartnoll *et al.* 1980). In brief, this research reported that while heroin-prescribed patients attended the clinic more regularly and showed some reduction in the extent of their criminal activity, nevertheless they showed no change in their other social activities, such as work, stable accommodation or diet, nor did they differ significantly in the physical complications of drug use from those denied such a prescription. These are all areas where proponents of legal prescribing of drugs of self-injection, then and now, believe there should be a harm reduction effect. While the majority of those who were refused a heroin prescription continued to inject illegally acquired supplies and only attended the clinic when they needed a specific service, a significant minority (one-fifth) of those refused heroin stabilized on oral methadone, and another one-fifth stopped all drug use. Although approximately two-thirds of both groups continued with some criminal activity the severity of this was, however, greater in those refused heroin, and this was reflected in a higher proportion of arrests and more time spent in custody (average of one week where heroin was prescribed and two weeks for those refused, during a twelve-month period).

In the context of this chapter on clinics, the reception that this research received in 1976 when presented to the staff of other clinics was as significant as the findings. The authors were clear and categorical that these findings could be regarded as a useful source of information on which to base more rational policies, and repeatedly stated that the findings were not a clear indication that one treatment was superior to the other. Nevertheless, research was perceived by many staff in London clinics as clear evidence for replacing injectable heroin maintenance with oral prescribing. In this author's opinion this probably reflected the already formulated clinical opinion that the policy of prescribing injectable drugs was, either or both, unhelpful to the patient and/or insupportable to therapeutically inclined staff. However, the research findings formed the focus for a prolonged debate between colleagues working within clinics and in street agencies. The latter by and large acknowledged that the continued prescribing of injectable drugs was not achieving significant change or harm reduction in the individual clients who attended their service. Following this debate many clinics made a considered decision in 1976/77 to move towards a more interventionist therapeutic approach with a refusal to prescribe injectable drugs to new patients.

Not just opiates

At the commencement and the end of the 1970s, the overwhelming majority of patients seen by drug clinics and street agencies were primarily dependent upon opioids. However, the majority were also secondary polydrug abusers (Bewley 1967; Hawkes *et al.* 1969; Mitcheson *et al.* 1970). There have been other periods before, during and after the 1970s when perhaps other drugs were more frequently used. For example, in the mid-1960s oral dexamphetamine (often stolen from manufacturers) had been a major primary drug of misuse. With increasing control the price of dexamphetamine tablets increased, and when in 1968 two independent doctors switched from prescribing cocaine to prescribing injectable methylamphetamine there was a fusing between members of the oral tablet culture and those with injection knowledge. When methylamphetamine was withdrawn from the retail pharmacy market by the manufacturer, in agreement with professional organizations, a proportion of these primary amphetamine users transferred to injecting methadone.

The injecting barbiturate epidemic

Next came the brief period of heavy misuse of methaqualone, under its trade name of Mandrax in 1968 (prior to the vogue for Quaaludes in the USA and Australia). This rapidly passed out of favour with intravenous drug users on account of its relative insolubility in water. The drug was also more strictly controlled under the Dangerous Drug Acts and it was replaced by the injection of barbiturates. Thus, during the early 1970s a combination of relatively easily available capsules of barbiturates, combined with the relative decrease in availability of injectable heroin as a result of clinic policies, the ending of the Vietnam War, and several years of drought in the Golden Triangle, facilitated the development of a primary barbiturate-injecting drug problem, especially in central London. Barbiturate capsules were so readily available from diverted pharmaceutical and prescription supplies, that attempts at controlled prescribing by clinics were rapidly abandoned in the face of continuing complications (for further exploration, see Chapter 6, Volume I, by Angela Burr).

Barbiturate misusers were frequently intoxicated, alternating with withdrawals typical of alcohol sedative withdrawals and often with *grand mal* epileptic fits occurring on clinic premises. Abscesses from intravenous injection were common, producing characteristic punched-out 'sterile' ulceration on the forearms and legs. Some users developed gangrene of hands and legs following accidental intra-arterial injection. The differential development of tolerance to the therapeutic or intoxicating dose on the one hand and to respiratory depression on the other, resulting in a narrowing of the therapeutic lethal ratio, gave rise to successive serious overdoses.

The inability of the out-patient clinics to assist the street agencies and hard-pressed accident and emergency departments of central London hospitals to cope with the casualties of this style of drug user, eventually resulted in the Department of Health funding a short-stay residential crisis intervention centre in London – known as City Roads. This service provided a welcome respite both to services concerned with intravenous barbiturate misuse and their clients. The CURB campaign, organized by the medical profession to reduce barbiturate prescribing, reduced availability of the drug on the black market. But the problem drug users did not fade away and City Roads had to modify its protocols in order to service the same rootless inner-city drug users, who were presenting the same acute medical and social problems but were now injecting relatively poor quality South-west Asian heroin which became available at the end of the 1970s.

Moving away from prescribing injectables

As indicated above, there was an initial drop in prescribing of heroin between 1967 and 1972 followed from 1976 by a further move away from injectable prescribing – see Figure 4.4 and Tables 4.1–4.4.

By the end of the decade there was a further modification of policy with an attempt to replace indefinite prescribing with contractual programmes. A limited stabilization period was followed by reducing prescriptions, linked contractually with the requirement to attend for either individual or group therapy targeted at individual change towards specific social changes and

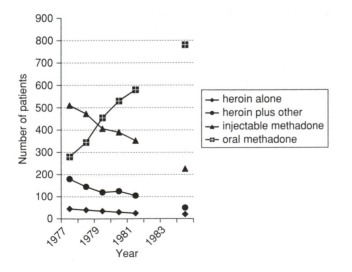

Figure 4.4 Number of patients receiving different drugs from all clinics in London
Source: As Figure 4.1.

Table 4.1 Heroin alone

Year	No. at clinics	No. receiving heroin alone	%	Average dose (mg)
1977	982	53	5	250
1978	962	47	5	219
1979	979	41	4	244
1980	1,037	38	4	249
1981	1,032	32	3	243
1984	1,081	23	2	181

Source: Previously unpublished data supplied by the London Consultants Group.

Table 4.2 Heroin with or without methadone (oral or injectable)

Year	No. at clinics	No. receiving heroin ± methadone	%	Average dose heroin	Average dose total opiate (mg)
1977	982	186	19	158	199
1978	962	148	15	142	178
1979	979	450	12	178	218
1980	1,037	121	12	150	189
1981	1,032	99	10	138	169
1984	1,081	59	5	130	170

Source: As Table 4.1.

Table 4.3 Injectable methadone with or without oral methadone (but not heroin)

Year	No. at clinics	No. receiving injectable ± oral methadone	%	Average injectable methadone	Average dose total opiate (mg)
1977	982	510	52	59	76
1978	962	473	49	59	69
1979	979	406	40	60	73
1980	1,037	390	38	63	78
1981	1,032	353	34	60	76
1984	1,081	226	21	49	69

Source: As Table 4.1.

a drug-free goal. It was the policy of many clinics to offer a series of such therapeutic interventions in the expectation that, over time, a significant proportion of drug users would accept such assistance towards a more stable and drug-free life. Certainly clinicians were not so naive to believe that the majority of patients would immediately stop drug use.

Table 4.4 Oral methadone alone

Year	No. at clinics	No. receiving oral methadone	%	Average dose (mg)
1977	982	286	29	39
1978	962	341	36	41
1979	979	451	46	37
1980	1,037	526	51	43
1981	1,032	578	56	48
1984	1,081	774	72	36

Source: As Table 4.1.

Diversity in the changes

The summated data in Tables 4.1 to 4.4 demonstrate a general overall policy change shared by the vast majority of London clinics, but there were, of course, exceptions. There always had been considerable variations between clinics in terms of the number of clients attending and their prescribing policies. Thus, for example, in 1977 the number of patients varied between 159 at the largest clinic and eight at the smallest. In the same year the percentage of clients receiving a heroin prescription varied from 0 per cent at a clinic with 89 patients and 1 per cent at the largest clinic then prescribing for 159, to 68 per cent of the 28 patients attending one of the smaller clinics. A clinic with 111 patients in 1977, of whom 48 per cent were receiving injectable prescriptions, had by 1979 144 patients, of whom only 20 per cent were receiving injectable prescriptions. That clinic's experience would suggest that a refusal to prescribe injectable drugs had not deterred patients from seeking help.

There were large variations in the average dose of heroin prescribed, which in part reflected the previous prescribing policy of that independent doctor who had transferred the initial group of patients to a particular clinic 10 years previously. The average dose of heroin in 1977 at the clinic with the highest proportion (68 per cent) of patients receiving heroin was 85 mg (range 10–150). In a larger clinic where 40 per cent were receiving heroin the mean daily dose was 224 mg (range 30–650) and another clinic recorded a top dose of 850 mg of heroin per day and a mean dose of 588 mg. By contrast the range of injectable methadone doses in 1979 was much smaller, individual doses ranged from 10 to 240 mg and clinic means ranged from 25 to 104 mg. For oral methadone the range was narrower still, with individual doses of between 1 and 200 mg and clinic means below 64 mg. Overall, therefore, while recognizing that the informal discussions at meetings induced movement towards a uniform practice, there were still very considerable variations both within and between clinics which were entirely at the clinical discretion of the staff concerned. See Figure 4.5 for a summary.

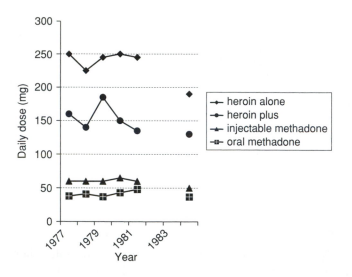

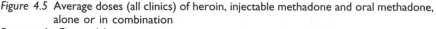

Figure 4.5 Average doses (all clinics) of heroin, injectable methadone and oral methadone, alone or in combination
Source: As Figure 4.1.

Why did the changes occur?

The changes during the 1970s were, in the main, a considered response by clinic workers who had acquired experience of the consequences of attempted stabilization with self-injectable prescriptions. Most of the clinics were anxious to continue to attract into a therapeutic environment those who could be assisted. There was concern that even when it was policy to offer a regular prescription of injectable drugs that there had generally been a lapse of 2 to 4 years between the time that someone was initiated into regular self-injection and the time they presented for treatment. Research into the epidemiology of syringe-transmitted hepatitis demonstrated that, by the time most patients presented for initial treatment, they had already been infected by syringe-transmitted hepatitis (Weller *et al.*, 1984). It was, therefore, felt that the correct emphasis was to develop outreach work and look to the availability of services and their image with the drug user, rather than rely on prescribing injectable drugs as a bait to bring in the customers.

It should be emphasized that at the time the changes in opioid prescribing were implemented there had not been a significant increase in the number of new patients presenting to clinics. The changes were based on clinical judgement in relation to the physical and social state of patients and their continued injection of a range of dangerous drugs. Increasing numbers of new referrals only began to present to treatment facilities at the end of the

1970s following the influx of South-west Asian heroin after the Iranian Revolution. The prior introduction of time-limited prescribing may, however, have subsequently enabled clinics to respond to the increased number of new referrals, without necessitating increasing staff and budgets. Although this chapter refers specifically to the 1970s it is appropriate to note that the additional funding provided from central government sources (first made available in 1984) was to cope with the increase in numbers presenting to clinics and particularly to enable services to be set up outside of London where illegal heroin was becoming increasingly available. Only a more recent increase in funding has been specifically linked to policy changes aimed at retaining patients in treatment for harm reduction in relation to reducing the spread of HIV through needle sharing.

Conclusion

The insistence that these changes were initiated on clinical judgement and not financial expediency is not a rhetorical argument. It is important to document and recall the experience of even the recent past. The uncontrolled prescribing of heroin by independent doctors between 1959 and 1968 was accompanied by a geometric increase in the number of new addicts to prescribed heroin, but a stable and low price for diverted heroin. The 1970s saw the erosion of the capacity of therapists to tolerate a numerically stable, but disorganized and distressing long-term regular clinic clientele who were persistent in their continued misuse of drugs, so that the clinics collectively swung the pendulum away from maintenance and towards confrontation of continued misuse of drugs, with active intervention and emphasis on facilitating change. Quite apart from the significant cost of funding prescriptions for long-term controlled stabilization, there is also a cost to be paid in terms of the burnout and disillusionment of dedicated staff, both in the statutory Community Drug Teams which have replaced the drug clinics, and in the non-statutory services which provide counselling and social support. The latter by and large acknowledged that the continued prescribing of injectable drugs was not achieving significant change or harm reduction in the individual clients who attend their service.

Clearly, the experience of the 1970s is highly relevant to the necessary continuing debate in the 1990s as to the appropriate form that drug services should take. It is tempting when confronted with an intractable problem to initiate radical changes in policy unsupported by systematic outcome studies. It is important therefore, first, to remember that a drug solution to the drug problem simply by prescribing injectable drugs is unlikely to be successful, and second that workers in drug services are not immune from the aphorism that 'the majority of the human race prefer the certainty of irrational conviction to the uncertainty of logical doubt'. There never has been, and never will be, a simple solution to the problem of substance misuse. And none of the range of services that must be provided comes cheap in terms of cash or human resources.

References

Bewley, T. H. (1965). *Lancet*, i, 808.
Bewley, T. H. (1967). *British Medical Journal*, 3, 603–5.
Brain Committee (Interdepartmental Committee on Drug Addiction, chaired by Sir Russell Brain) (1965). Second report. HMSO, London.
Connell, P. H. (1991). Treatment of drug dependent patients 1968–69. *British Journal of Addiction*, 86, 913–90.
Dole, V. P., Nysvander, M. E. and Kreek, M. J. (1966). Narcotic blockade. *Archives of Internal Medicine*, 118, 304–9.
Dorn, N. and South, N. (1985). *Helping drug users*. Gower, Aldershot.
Hartnoll, R., Mitcheson, M., Battersby, A., Brown, G., Ellis, M., Fleming, P. and Hedley, N. (1980). Evaluation of heroin maintenance in controlled trial. *Archives of General Psychiatry*, 37, 877–84.
Hawkes, D., Mitcheson, M., Ogborne, A. and Edwards, G. (1969). Abuse of methylamphetamine. *British Medical Journal*, 2, 715–21.
Larrimore, G. W. and Brill, H. (1967). Epidemiological factors in drug addiction in England and USA. *Public Health Reports*, 11, 555–60.
Mitcheson, M. C. and Hartnoll, R. L. (1978). Conflicts in deciding treatment within drug dependency clinics. In *Problems of drug abuse in Britain* (ed. D. J. West), pp. 74–7. Cambridge University Institute of Criminology.
Mitcheson, M. C., Davidson, J., Hawkes, D., Hitchens, L. and Molone, S. (1970). Sedative abuse by heroin addicts. *Lancet*, i, 606–7.
Schur, E. M. (1963). *Narcotic addiction in Britain and America*. Tavistock, London.
Stimson, G. V. (1973). *Heroin and behaviour: diversity among addicts attending London clinics*. Irish University Press, Shannon, Ireland.
Weller, I. V. D., Cohn, D., Sierralta, A., Mitcheson, M., Ross, M. G. R., Montano, L., Scheuer, P. and Thomas, H. L. (1984). Clinical, biochemical, histological, and ultrastructural features of liver disease in drug abusers. *Gut*, 25, 417–23.

Chapter 5

The fall and rise of the general practitioner

Alan Glanz

(This chapter originally appeared in J. Strang and M. Gossop (eds) *Heroin Addiction and Drug Policy: The British System*, Oxford University Press, 1994.)

A constant theme in the evolution of the British system during the twentieth century has been the shifting balance in policy and service provision between the roles of the specialist and the generalist in responding to drug misusers. Over this period the position of the general medical practitioner (GP) has undergone major transitions as policy has developed in response to perceived changes in the character of the drugs problem. Several distinct phases are identifiable, during which the GP first becomes established in addiction treatment, then is displaced by the specialist, and finally re-emerges in a key role. These changes in the role of the GP in the treatment of drug misuse can also be viewed against the background of changes in the standing of the GP within the wider system of medical care.

Emergence of the GP in addiction treatment

The role of GPs in the treatment of drug misuse emerged with the disease concept of narcotic addiction in the latter part of the nineteenth century. It has been suggested that the elaboration of the disease theory of addiction and treatment structures was part of the process of professional self-affirmation on the part of a medical profession gaining in confidence and prestige (Berridge and Edwards 1981). By this time the GP was a well-established medical figure. While its precise origins are uncertain, it has been established that the term GP was unknown before 1800, came into use increasingly between 1810 and 1830 and was firmly established by 1840 when GPs formed over 80 per cent of the medical profession (Loudon 1983). These GPs arose to meet a demand from the growing middle classes of Victorian Britain for a personal or family doctor.

It was morphine habituation among the middle classes rather than opium consumption among the lower classes that formed the clinical basis of the disease theory of addiction, for its formulation and application was limited to the class of patients doctors were likely to treat at this time (Berridge 1979). No consensus was established, however, on the best method of treatment. In general the role of the GP was to devise and supervise a gradual withdrawal regime. The method implemented varied widely and for certain cases involved institutional care.

In the early part of the twentieth century the system of medical management of addiction was threatened by the extension to the civilian population of the drug control regulations covering members of the armed forces which were passed during the First World War. Possession of opiate drugs and cocaine was restricted to authorized persons. Under regulations of the Dangerous Drugs Act of 1920, a medical practitioner was authorized to possess and supply drugs only so far as was necessary for the practice of his profession (Bean 1974).

Some GPs with addict patients interpreted this as permitting them to 'continue prescribing regular maintenance doses'. However, the Home Office was not satisfied with this situation and wanted to restrict the scope for interpretation of the Act. In order to secure an authoritative statement on the professional legitimacy of supplying opiate drugs to addicts, a committee chaired by Sir Humphrey Rolleston was appointed in 1924 (Berridge 1984). The Committee's Report of 1926 is a landmark in the evolution of British policy on addiction, forming the basis of the 'British System' (Departmental Committee 1926). The recommendations of the Report were implemented under further regulations of the Dangerous Drug Act. The approach adopted by the Rolleston Committee – composed entirely of medical men – rested squarely on their acceptance of the disease nature of addiction. The outcome amounted essentially to the preservation of the right of medical practitioners to prescribe opiate drugs not only for withdrawal treatment but also in 'non-diminishing doses' for certain patients. The case for the prescribing role of the medical practitioner was made by the Committee on grounds of patient welfare, but the impulse to protect professional medical control also played a part (Berridge 1980).

It is worth noting the contrast with the contemporary scene in the USA. As Trebach has shown, the Harrison Act of 1914 contained very similar language to the Dangerous Drugs Act in restricting dispensation of controlled drugs by a doctor to the 'course of his professional practice only'. The difference was in the interpretation of this phrase in the USA where a large number of doctors were prosecuted during the 1920s for prescribing to addicts as this was viewed as beyond the scope of their legitimate role (Trebach 1982).

For some 40 years the position of the GP in the treatment system established by the Rolleston Committee remained undisturbed. Over this period British society underwent profound social changes and the social structure of the drugs scene underwent a transformation of its own. The addicts of the Rolleston era were never likely to constitute a social problem. They were a relatively small number of largely professional and middle-class individuals who formed no kind of social network. By the mid-1960s the social circles of doctors and addicts, which in the Rolleston era had to some extent over-lapped, now became firmly detached and distant from each other as the social characteristics of drug users were rapidly changing. The consequence was a radical restructuring of the treatment system and the effective removal of the GP from the treatment system.

Removal of the GP from addiction treatment

Some awareness of emerging changes in the drugs scene is registered by the appointment in 1958 of an Interdepartmental Committee on Drug Addiction under the chairmanship of Sir Russell Brain. The conclusion of the Committee's Report in 1961 was that the Rolleston system should remain intact as there was no evidence that the right of doctors to provide drugs of addiction in the treatment of addict patients had led to any increase in the number of addicts (Interdepartmental Committee 1961).

However, the changing nature of the drugs scene could not be ignored for long. In 1954 there were 57 known heroin addicts and in 1959 there were 68, but by 1964 there were 342 heroin addicts known to the Home Office (Spear 1969). The Brain Committee was reconvened in 1964 specifically to consider the need for revising policy on the prescribing of addictive drugs. The Committee's Report identified the source of the unprecedented growth in addiction as 'the activity of a very few doctors who have prescribed excessively for addicts' (Interdepartmental Committee 1965).

The solution which the Committee recommended was to circumscribe for the first time the ability of medical practitioners to prescribe drugs according to their own professional judgement. The Dangerous Drugs Act of 1967 gave legislative effect to the Committee proposals. The power to prescribe heroin and cocaine in the treatment of addiction was removed from ordinary medical practitioners and placed in the hands of doctors granted a special licence from the Home Office. These doctors were very largely consultant psychiatrists in charge of hospital-based special centres which were now set up to treat addicts.

The incursion into clinical autonomy represented by the proposals of the Second Brain Committee was greeted with protests by some sections of the medical profession. In particular a Working Party of the British Medical Association (BMA), a body mainly representing the interests of GPs, was highly critical (Smart 1985). These objections were not, however, vigorously pursued. As Smart has noted, the BMA made it clear that drug addicts were not popular patients and GPs were probably glad to be relieved of the responsibility for dealing with them (Smart 1985). The restriction on prescribing did not apply to supply of heroin for medical treatment other than addiction. The curtailment of clinical freedom was thus accepted.

It is apparent that to a certain extent doctors treating addicts were being made scapegoats for a problem which was emerging as the result of far more complex social forces. A leading article in the *British Medical Journal* complaining at the threat to clinical freedom contained in the Committee's recommendations certainly had a point in arguing that it was 'a grave step to take in – it would appear – to control the over-prescribing habits of only a handful of doctors' (British Medical Journal 1965).

The establishment of a new treatment system towards the end of the 1960s was linked to a new understanding of the nature of the drugs problem. While, as in the Rolleston period, addicts remained an individually isolated set of mainly middle-class and therapeutically addicted persons, it was appropriate that treatment should remain in the hands of individual general and private medical practitioners. When addiction came to be seen, in the words of the second Brain Committee, as a 'socially infectious disease', with the heroin users now constituting a distinct subculture within society, individual medical practitioners no longer offered an adequate response. The system needed to be strengthened. The new addiction treatment centre, located within a hospital framework and staffed by a multidisciplinary team headed by a consultant psychiatrist, was far less vulnerable to the pressure and demands of addicts. As Stimson and Oppenheimer (1982) have put it: 'The new element introduced in the rethinking of policy in the 1960s was the emphasis on the social control of addiction.'

The decline of general practice within medicine

The removal of the GP from the addiction treatment system can also be set within the context of developments in the status of general practice within the wider system of medicine.

Throughout the 1920s and 1930s there was a rapid acceleration of a process of change within medicine that had already been under way during the nineteenth century. The 'division of medicine' – the separation of general practice from hospital care – accentuated, with hospital medicine becoming increasingly dominant (Honigsbaum 1979). Advances in medical knowledge, in diagnostics and laboratory-based investigations, and in technological applications in treatment meant that specialization became inevitable (Stevens 1966). A number of long-standing functions of the GP were transferred to hospital-based specialists. The status of the GP declined.

During the 1950s and most of the 1960s general practice remained an unattractive career option for qualifying doctors. National surveys of medical students in 1961 and in 1966 showed that only around one-quarter of final-year students gave general practice as their first choice of career (Martin 1984). Indeed, the total number of GPs was declining and so was the ratio

of GPs to patients (Jefferys and Sachs 1983). The view of the medical establishment was summed up in the statement in 1966 of Lord Moran, President
of the Royal College of Physicians, that general practice medicine was an
occupation for those who 'fall off the ladder' and failed to become specialists
(Hart 1988). GPs themselves complained that they were operating merely as
signposts to the specialists, wasting their training on attending to trivialities
rather than doing 'real medicine' (Cartwright 1967). The mid-1960s probably represented the nadir of general practice within the medical system.
It was in this climate that the new hospital-based specialist addiction treatment infrastructure was devised, which effectively eliminated the GPs from
the system.

The reinstatement of the GP in addiction treatment

The creation of the specialist hospital-based addiction treatment centres
together with the licensing system effectively marginalized the role of the
GP in addiction treatment for more than a decade. It is unlikely that substantial numbers of GPs had in any case been involved in treating the
metropolitan concentration of addicts in the 1960s. The effect, however, was
to limit the variety of treatment opportunities as the drugs problem evolved
during the 1970s and the drug clinics remained a largely monopolistic and
somewhat monolithic service for addicts.

There was some awareness during this period that addicts were seeking
alternatives to what they regarded as narrow prescribing policies practised
by the drug clinics. The private practitioner emerged as the 'unacceptable
face' of addiction treatment (Bewley *et al.* 1975; Bewley and Ghodse 1983).
The opiate-focused hospital treatment centres lacked the flexibility to respond
to the developing drugs problem characterized by polydrug abuse involving barbiturates, tranquillizers, amphetamines and opiates (Lancet 1979).
Private and general practitioners, together with voluntary drug agencies,
were increasingly in contact with drug misusers whose treatment needs or
demands left them outside the clinic system.

However, it was the rapid change in the scale of drugs problem rather
than changes in its form which led, by the early 1980s, to the return of the
GP as a major agent in the treatment framework. This re-entry of the GP
was first recognized at an official level in the 1982 Report on Treatment and
Rehabilitation from the Advisory Council in the Misuse of Drugs (ACMD).
The ACMD had been established under the 1968 and 1971 Misuse of Drugs
Act as an independent committee of experts serviced by the Home Office.
Their 1982 Report noted, 'the fact that over the last few years an increasing
proportion of drug misusers is being treated not in the hospital based treatment clinics, but by doctors in general practice (both NHS and private)' and
referred to this as 'an unplanned development' (ACMD 1982). The ACMD
raised the issue of the role of GPs as a policy question for the first time since

the second Brain Committee Report of 1965. According to the ACMD – in some respects echoing the Brain Committee – the principal problem of this 'unplanned development' was the 'extent to which controlled drugs are prescribed injudiciously' (ACMD 1982). Of course GPs were still entitled to prescribe any drugs, including opiates other than heroin and excluding cocaine, in the treatment of drug dependence.

The ACMD expressed concern about a number of aspects of the GPs' position in relation to drug-taking patients – their lack of specialized knowledge and limited training opportunities, their relative isolation leaving them vulnerable to pressure from drug misusers, and inadequate access to support staff and appropriate facilities for full patient assessment. Nevertheless, the ACMD was prepared, providing there were 'strict safeguards', to accept 'a possible role for some doctors outside the specialist services to play a part in the treatment of problem drug takers' (ACMD 1982).

The subject of safeguards regarding prescribing was soon tackled by the issue to all doctors in 1984 of 'Guidelines of good clinical practice in the treatment of drug misuse', drawn up by a Medical Working Group on Drug Dependence set up by the Department of Health in response to the recommendations of the ACMD Report (Medical Working Group 1984). The guidelines expressed encouragement to GPs 'to play a major role', and stated that 'it is the responsibility of all doctors to provide care for both the general health needs and drug related problems' of drug misusers (Medical Working Group 1984).

Clearly policy was now about reinstating the GP as a key actor in the response to drug misuse. In 1985 the Minister of State with responsibility for drugs policy expressed the view that it was the 'duty' of every GP to provide a service for drug misusers (Social Services Committee 1985). A Health Circular on services for drug misusers issued in 1986 by the Department of Health described the Department's policy as encouraging GPs 'to play a major part in the care and treatment of drug misusers' (Department of Health 1986).

In what circumstances did this fundamental shift in policy come about? The answer can be indicated by contrasting the introductions to two government publications on the prevention and treatment of drug misuse issued six years apart. The earlier document of 1979 stated that 'the United Kingdom appears at present to have a relatively stable situation as far as narcotic dependence is concerned' (Central Office of Information 1979). The second in 1985 stated by contrast that 'In Britain . . . the rapid rise in the misuse of drugs . . . has emerged as one of the most serious social problems of the 1980s' (Central Office of Information 1985). The statistics on addicts notified by all doctors to the Home Office illustrate this dramatic change in the dimensions of the British drugs problem: 1979, 2,385 addicts notified; 1985, 8,819 addicts notified (Home Office 1989). These figures reflect the rapid spread of heroin use among young people in diverse areas of the country. For many of these young people a hospital treatment centre was inaccessibly distant or the waiting time for an appointment was unacceptably long as the prevalence of drug misuse outstripped the capacity of the specialist services to respond.

The GP, on the other hand, is an accessible and to many a natural source to turn to for help. The growth in the involvement of GPs is also illustrated by Home Office statistics. In 1970 GPs were responsible for 15 per cent of notifications made by all doctors, in 1975 for 29 per cent and in 1984 for 55 per cent (ACMD 1982; Home Office 1989). An indication of the extent of GP involvement was provided by the results of a national survey of GPs in mid-1985, showing that about one in five GPs throughout England and Wales would see at least one opiate drug misuser in a given four-week period and GPs as a whole would deal with some 40,000 new cases of opiate drug misuse over a twelve-month period (Glanz and Taylor 1986).

Policy in the early and mid-1980s reflected the urgent need to respond to the growing drugs problem. GPs were now seen as a valuable resource in strengthening the framework for managing that problem.

The changing ideological context of policy

In respect of the role of GPs, the policy response to an escalating drugs problem in the early and mid-1980s was clearly very different from the response to that of the early and mid-1960s. The ideological context of drugs policy formation had changed significantly.

Within the drugs field a change had occurred over this period in the definition of the problem at which policy was directed. The earlier disease-based notion of addiction gave way to the notion of 'problem drug taking' as formulated by the ACMD in its 1982 Report Treatment and rehabilitation. The idea of the problem drug taker involves a broader perspective, moving away from a substance focus and recognizing the personal, social and medical (including dependence) difficulties which may be associated with use of a range of drugs (ACMD 1982). This reconceptualization of the drugs problem offers scope for professionals other than drug dependence specialists to play a role.

Linked to this formulation of the problem drug taker is the perception of the 'normalization' of the drug misuser. Heroin and other drug use in the 1980s was on a far greater scale and had a wider geographical distribution than in the 1960s. From the point of view of service provision, the implication is that 'as notorious drugs (such as use of heroin) become more widespread in a population the people using them are likely to be more normal (statistically and in other senses) than the abnormal population who presented originally' (Strang 1984). As a consequence, the view that drug misusers need to be dealt with by specialists is undermined: 'if some of the drug-takers are becoming more normal, then perhaps some of the drug services should do likewise' (Strang 1989).

A further element in the changing ideological context of policy is the rise of the 'community' response to drug problems (Stimson 1987). As in the wider field of health and social services, provision of drug misuse services in the 1980s had been developing a community care approach, aiming to deal with the individual's problems within the social setting which they inhabit rather than offer an institutional response. 'Community drug teams' have been widely established, as in the 'model service' in the North Western Regional Health Authority (Strang 1989). These multidisciplinary groups operate outside of institutional frameworks to facilitate direct access to help and work to mobilize generic services in the community, particularly GPs, to respond to drug problems. (See also Chapters 6, 7 and 8, this volume.)

The rise of general practice within medicine

These changes in the construction of the nature of the drugs problem and its management have promoted the GP to a prominent position as a focus for policy development and service planning. To some extent the shifts in the drugs field described above have been special applications of broader developments in health and social care. The trend towards community care and 'de-institutionalization' has had a wide impact on service provision; for example, in the case of alcohol services where the problem orientation (rather than substance orientation) initially developed (Stockwell and Clement 1987). The role of GP was widely enhanced by these developments. Indeed, the status of general practice had been rising steadily for some years.

Leaders within general practice had been aware for many years of the need to rebuild a sense of professional self-esteem. General practice slowly but successfully established its credentials as a speciality in its own right following the publication of the Report of the Royal Commission on Medical Education (Royal Commission on Medical Education 1968), with medical schools setting up academic departments of general practice and vocational training becoming mandatory (in 1982) for entry into general practice (Wilkin et al. 1987).

Cognitive foundations for the professional development of general practice required a specialist body of knowledge for a distinct specialism. This emerged with the formulation of an alternative model of medicine to that of hospital medicine, the approach of 'biographical medicine' (Armstrong 1979). Here the emphasis is on the patient as a whole, and an interpretation of signs and symptoms is given in the context of the patient's biography and environment. The holistic approach was represented in the widely influential work of Balint, who identified a particular role for the GP in dealing with the many patients presenting with symptoms which apparently had no organic basis (Balint 1966).

The increased self-confidence of general practice was supported by and reflected in improvements in conditions of service, the growth of large group practices and health centres, and the emergence of the primary health-care team. In contrast to the position in the 1960s, by 1984 general practice had become the most popular career choice of British medical students (Lancet 1984). Thus, the whole position of general practice had been vastly strengthened and the GP could meaningfully be called upon to play a significant role in the treatment of drug misuse.

The advent of AIDS and the future role of the GP

The threat of human immunodeficiency virus (HIV) and acquired immune deficiency syndrome (AIDS) associated with use of contaminated injecting equipment has brought general practice even more firmly into a key position in the strategy for responding to drug problems. According to the first AIDS and Drug Misuse Report of the ACMD, 'the network of general practitioners offers an unrivalled system of health care provision with great opportunities for intervention with drug misusing patients' (ACMD 1988). The Report noted, however, that the opportunities for GP intervention 'have not yet been adequately seized', and went on to emphasize that 'the advent of HIV makes it essential that all GPs should provide care and advice for drug misusing patients to help them move away from behaviour which may result in them acquiring and spreading the virus' (ACMD 1988).

The extent to which GPs will respond to the challenge of HIV in the context of drug misuse is at the present moment an open question. There is no doubt that GPs remain widely involved with drug misusers. Home Office figures show that a total of 7,947 addicts were notified by GPs during 1989, representing 54 per cent of notifications from all doctors (Home Office 1990). Furthermore, a survey of 10 per cent of all GPs in England and Wales undertaken in early 1990 found that an estimated 19,000 drug misusers – covering use by injection and by other routes of heroin, other opiates, cocaine/crack or amphetamines, and use by injection of other drugs – are currently under the care of GPs, with around one in four GPs having at least one drug misuser currently under their care (Glanz and Friendship 1990). However, despite this extensive contact, evidence from several studies indicates that GPs are not responding with enthusiasm to the prospects of working with drug misuser patients.

The model extensively promoted in the North Western Regional Health Authority in which GPs and general psychiatrists were encouraged to provide the bulk of services to drug misusers, with specialists operating as sources of advice and teaching, has been deemed a qualified failure by those who implemented and monitored the policy (Strang 1991; Strang et al. 1991, 1992). The conclusion they draw from this experience is that the likely effectiveness of such a strategy for combating HIV infection in drug misusers (which presumes that a widespread contribution will be forthcoming from the generalist, in particular the GP) must be open to considerable doubt (Donmall *et al.* 1990; Strang *et al.* 1991; Strang 1991).

Studies of the role of the GP in relation to broad issues and of HIV and AIDS have found the area of drug misuse to be particularly problematic. A survey of two groups of GPs, one group of GP trainers and one non-trainer GPs, found that both groups were reluctant to care for intravenous drug misusers and that the drug abuse problems of many patients were seen as the single greatest deterrent to caring for AIDS (Sibbald and Freeling 1988). An interview study among London GPs concerning management of problems relating to HIV found that over one-quarter would not accept known intra-venous drug users as patients and a further 11 per cent would accept them only under defined conditions (King 1989). In the Parkside Health District in London a recent survey found that only 29 per cent of the GPs in the area were willing to care for HIV antibody-positive intravenous drug users, com-pared with 60 per cent willing to care for heterosexuals and 47 per cent for homosexuals with HIV (Roderick *et al.* 1990).

Findings from the 1990 national postal questionnaire survey referred to above, covering a 10 per cent random sample of GPs in England and Wales, throw some light on the prospects for GP involvement with drug misusers (Glanz and Friendship 1990). Just under one-half (47 per cent) of GPs agreed that they would undertake treatment of drug misusers as willingly as they would any other type of patient in need of care, while 41 per cent disagreed with this position. Many GPs are prepared only to have a minimal involvement – 43 per cent agreed that they would refer any patient consulting for drug misuse to a specialist service and make no further appointment to see the patient for this problem. On the other hand, 80 per cent agreed that they were willing to collaborate with a specialist service in joint management of drug misusers.

In its Report on AIDS and drug misuse the ACMD stated that 'the spread of HIV is a greater danger to individual and public health than drug misuse' and hence there was a need 'to work with those who continue to misuse drugs to help them reduce the risks involved in doing so, above all the risk of acquiring or spreading HIV' (ACMD 1988). To what extent would GPs accept this role? The findings of the national survey are that 39 per cent of GPs expressed agreement and 41 per cent disagreement in respect of their own willingness to work with drug misusers in this way (Glanz and Friend-ship 1990).

A further recommendation of the ACMD is that 'all GPs should accept their responsibility for the ongoing health care of drug misusers with HIV disease' (ACMD 1989). In the national survey just under two-thirds (63 per cent) were in agreement that they would be willing to do this, with one-fifth (21 per cent) disagreeing. However, the relative aversiveness of drug misusers as patients in this context emerges in the finding that only about one-half of GPs (53 per cent) agreed that they would accept on to their list an HIV antibody-positive drug misuser as willingly as they would any other HIV antibody-positive patient seeking care, while 30 per cent disagreed (Glanz and Friendship 1990).

The national survey clearly revealed that GPs hold a range of negative opinions about drug misusers. Most GPs believe that drug misusers would present more severe management problems than any other type of patient (79 per cent), would make unmanageable demands on their time (71 per cent), and would not comply with any treatment regimen (55 per cent). Furthermore, GPs feel that working with drug misusers was unlikely to be rewarded by satisfying results (62 per cent) and would expose them and others in the surgery to aggressive and threatening behaviour (73 per cent) (Glanz and Friendship 1990). It may be the case that there is a fundamental difficulty for the GP in dealing with patients who apparently violate so many of the standard expectations of the doctor–patient relationship (McKeganey and Boddy 1988).

The imperative of AIDS prevention requires GPs to perform a more demanding role than previously. The new model for the GP has been set out by Robertson, describing an Edinburgh general practice: 'our own policy revolves around the philosophy of risk reduction and therefore prescribing becomes a device used if it is seen as a method of prevention of greater dangers' (Robertson 1989). This involves an assessment of the complex options opened up by the 'hierarchy of goals' approach elaborated by the ACMD (1988). Such an approach would perhaps require the GP to undertake a more sophisticated assessment and response than that described for a standardized methadone detoxification regimen (Medical Working Group 1984).

Local evidence suggests that the prescribing option in the context of risk reduction will not be readily taken up. In a survey in one inner London area, only 15 per cent of GPs were prepared to undertake methadone withdrawal and 10 per cent methadone maintenance of narcotic users (Bell et al. 1990). The 1990 national survey shows that GPs do not regard themselves as properly equipped to handle these patients – only 15 per cent agreed that their knowledge of the clinical aspects of drug misuse was sufficient for meeting the needs of patients who may present with this problem (Glanz and Friendship 1990). Indeed, Robertson and colleagues have themselves revealed the extent of the burden which drug misusers might place on GP services. They found from an analysis of practice records over a two-year period in 1986–87 that a sample of 25 HIV antibody-positive drug misusers made a total of 1,485 surgery visits and that a second sample of 25 non-HIV drug misusers made a total of 1,130 visits (Roberts et al. 1989).

If GPs are to be recruited to a sustained involvement with drug misusers in the AIDS era it is vital to guard against the phenomenon observed in the course of the heroin 'epidemic' in the Wirral area of north-west England in the early 1980s, in which, after initial high levels of involvement, GP 'burn-out' led to their wholesale disengagement from treating heroin-user patients (Parker *et al.* 1988). One possible way of sustaining the involvement of GPs would be to offer a financial incentive for treating these patients – a proposal which the ACMD (1988) recommended should be explored. Indeed, one GP with experience of drug misusers argued that a small payment for each drug misuser treated per year would be a very cost-effective inducement to GPs and would 'achieve a substantial increase in the nation's drug treatment workforce' (Waller 1990). However, such an approach certainly has considerable cost – and ethical – implications, and its potential effectiveness is open to doubt. In the 1990 national survey, only about one-quarter of GPs (27 per cent) agreed that some financial incentive would encourage them to extend their involvement with drug misusers.

How can GPs be effectively encouraged to overcome the numerous obstacles they identify as inhibiting their willingness to work with drug misusers? The national survey points to several possible approaches. One-half of GPs in the survey agreed that provision of training opportunities in the management of drug misuse would encourage them to extend their involvement with these patients. The availability of further human resources would be an equal incentive for GPs. About one-half of GPs (49 per cent) agreed that additional staffing resources for the primary health-care team would encourage them to extend their involvement with drug misusers.

The most effective strategy for promoting GP involvement emerging from the 1990 national survey is the provision of greater access to specialist back-up services. More than two-thirds of GPs (68 per cent) agreed that this would encourage them to extend their involvement with drug misusers. This fits with the finding reported above of the very high proportion of GPs in the survey (80 per cent) who expressed willingness to collaborate with specialist services in joint management of drug misusers.

Conclusion

The future role of the GP within the system of provision for drug misusers is an uncertain one. The changes in policy which have brought about the fall and rise of the GP in this system have been, like so much of drug policy, largely reactive and pragmatic rather than planned and strategic. The current policy of promoting GP involvement has not been implemented within a framework of specific measures designed to secure favourable conditions for a successful outcome. Indeed recent developments in broader health service policy concerning the contractual responsibilities of GPs may have a counterproductive effect in this respect (Robertson and Witcombe 1990). For GPs, HIV adds a new complication to the already difficult task of dealing with drug misusers, and yet at the same time their role within the system of provision becomes more significant than ever before. Without active steps to secure their involvement the next phase in the history of the role of GPs in the treatment of drug misuse is likely to be one of detachment and disengagement.

References

ACMD (Advisory Council on the Misuse of Drugs) (1982). Treatment and rehabilitation. HMSO, London.

ACMD (1988). AIDS and drug misuse. Part 1. HMSO, London.

ACMD (1989). AIDS and drug misuse. Part 2. HMSO, London.

Armstrong, D. (1979). The emancipation of biographical medicine. *Social Science and Medicine*, 13, 1–8.

Balint, M. (1966). *The doctor, his patient, and the illness*. Pitman, London.

Bean, P. (1974). *The social control of drugs*. Martin Robertson, London.

Bell, G., Cohen, J. and Cremona, A. (1990). How willing are general practitioners to manage narcotic misuse? *Health Trends*, 22 (2), 56–7.

Berridge, V. (1979). Morality and medical science: concepts of narcotic addiction in Britain, 1820–1926. *Annals of Science*, 36, 67–85.

Berridge, V. (1980). The making of the Rolleston Report, 1908–1926. *Journal of Drug Issues*, Winter, pp. 7–28.

Berridge, V. (1984). Drugs and social policy in the establishment of drug control in Britain, 1900–1930. *British Journal of Addiction*, 79, 17–29.

Berridge, V. and Edwards, G. (1981). *Opium and the people: opiate use in nineteenth-century England*. Croom Helm, London.

Bewley, T. H. and Ghodse, A. H. (1983). Unacceptable face of private practice: prescription of controlled drugs to addicts. *British Medical Journal*, 286, 1876–7.

Bewley, T. H., Teggin, A. F., Mahon, T. A. and Webb, D. (1975). Conning the general practitioner – how drug abusing patients obtain prescriptions. *Journal of the Royal College of General Practitioners*, 25, 654–7.

Brain Committee (1965). See Interdepartmental Committee (1965).

British Medical Journal (1965). Control of drug addiction. *British Medical Journal*, 2, 1259–60.

Cartwright, A. (1967). *Patients and their doctors: a study of general practice*. Routledge, London.

Central Office of Information (1979). *The prevention and treatment of drug misuse in Britain*. HMSO, London.

Central Office of Information (1985). *The prevention and treatment of drug misuse in Britain*. Central Office of Information, London.

Department of Health (1986). *Health Service development. Services for drug misusers*. Health Circular HC(86)3.

Departmental Committee (1926). Report. Departmental Committee on Morphine and Heroin Addiction. HMSO, London.

Donmall, M. C., Webster, A., Strang, J. and Tantam, D. (1990). The introduction of community-based services for drug misusers: impact and outcome in the North-West, 1982–1986. Report to the Department of Health, England. (Available from ISDD (Institute for the Study of Drug Dependence) Library, London.)

Glanz, A. and Taylor, C. (1986). Findings of a national survey of the role of general practitioners in the treatment of opiate misuse: extent of contact. *British Medical Journal*, 293, 427–30.

Glanz, A. and Friendship, C. (1990). The role of general practitioners in the treatment of drug misuse. Findings from a survey of GPs in England and Wales, 1989. Report to the Department of Health (unpublished).

Hart, J. T. (1988). *A new kind of doctor*. Merlin, London.

Home Office (1989). Statistics of drug addicts notified to the Home Office, UK 1988. Statistical Bulletin 13/89. Home Office, London.

Home Office (1990). Statistics of the misuse of drugs: addicts notified to the Home Office, UK 1989. Statistical Bulletin 7/90. Home Office, London.

Honigsbaum, F. (1979). *The division in British medicine: a history of the separation of general practice from hospital care 1911–1968*. Kogan Page, London.

Interdepartmental Committee (1961). Report. Interdepartmental Committee on Drug Addiction. HMSO, London.

Interdepartmental Committee (1965). Second Report. Interdepartmental Committee on Drug Addiction. HMSO, London.

Jefferys, M. and Sachs, H. (1983). *Rethinking general practice: dilemmas in primary medical care*. Tavistock, London.

King, M. B. (1989). Psychological and social problems of HIV infection: interviews with general practitioners in London. *British Medical Journal*, 299, 713–17.

Lancet (1979). Drug addiction: time for reappraisal. *Lancet*, ii, 289–90.

Lancet (1984). Towards better general practice. *Lancet*, ii, 1436–8.

Loudon, I. S. L. (1983). The origins of the general practitioner. *Journal of the Royal College of General Practitioners*, 33, 13–18.

Martin, F. M. (1984). *Between the Acts: community mental health services 1959–1983*. Nuffield Provincial Hospitals Trust, London.

McKeganey, N. P. and Boddy, F. A. (1988). General practitioners and opiate abusing patients. *Journal of the Royal College of General Practitioners*, 38, 73–5.

Medical Working Group (1984). Guidelines of good clinical practice in the treatment of drug misuse. Report of the Medical Working Group on Drug Dependence. Department of Health, London.

Parker, H., Bakx, K. and Newcombe, R. (1988). *Living with heroin*. Open University Press, Milton Keynes.

Roberts, J. J. K., Skidmore, C. A. and Robertson, J. R. (1989). Human immunodeficiency virus in drug misusers and increased consultation rate in general practice. *Journal of the Royal College of General Practitioners*, 39, 373–4.

Robertson, J. R. (1989). Treatment of drug misuse in the general practice setting. *British Journal of Addiction*, 84, 377–80.

Robertson, R. and Witcombe, J. (1990). Drug problems and primary health care. *British Journal of Addiction*, 85, 685–6.

Roderick, P., Victor, C. R. and Beardow, R. (1990). Developing care in the community: GPs and the HIV epidemic. *AIDS Care*, 2, 127–32.

Royal Commission on Medical Education (1968). Report. HMSO, London.

Sibbald, B. and Freeling, P. (1988). AIDS and the future general practitioner. *Journal of the Royal College of General Practitioners*, 38, 500–2.

Smart, C. (1985). Social policy and drug dependence: an historical case study. *Drug and Alcohol Dependence*, 16, 169–80.

Social Services Committee (1985). Misuse of drugs. Fourth Report from the House of Commons Social Services Committee. HMSO, London.

Spear, H. B. (1969). The growth of heroin addiction in the UK. *British Journal of Addiction*, 64, 245.

Stevens, R. (1966). *Medical practice in modern England: the impact of specialisation and state medicine*. Yale University Press, New Haven.

Stimson, G. V. (1987). British drug policies in the 1980s: a preliminary analysis and suggestions for research. *British Journal of Addiction*, 82, 477–88.

Stimson, G. V. and Oppenheimer, E. (1982). *Heroin addiction: treatment and control in Britain*. Tavistock, London.

Stockwell, T. and Clement, S. (eds) (1987). *Helping the problem drinker: new initiatives in community care*. Croom Helm, London.

Strang, J. (1984). Changing the image of the drug taker. *Health and Social Service Journal*, 11 October, 1202–4.

Strang, J. (1989). A model service: turning the generalist on to drugs. In *Drugs and British society* (ed. S. MacGregor), pp. 143–69. Routledge, London.

Strang, J. (1991). Service development and organisation: drugs. In *International handbook on addiction behaviour* (ed. I. Glass), pp. 283–91. Routledge, London.

Strang, J., Donmall, M. C., Webster, A., Abbey, J. and Tantam, D. (1991). A bridge not far enough: Community Drug Teams and doctors in the North Western Region, 1982–1986 (Research monograph no. 3). Institute for the Study of Drug Dependence (ISDD), London.

Strang, J., Smith, M. and Spurrell, S. (1992). Community. Drug Team: goals, methods and activity analysis. *British Journal of Addiction*, 87, 169–78.

Trebach, A. (1982). *The heroin solution*. Yale University Press, New Haven.

Waller, T. (1990). Ways to open the surgery door. *Druglink*, 5 (3), 10–11.

Wilkin, D., Hallam, L., Leavey, R. and Metcalfe, D. (1987). *Anatomy of urban general practice*. Tavistock, London.

Chapter 6

The GP and the drug misuser in the new NHS

A new 'British System'

Clare Gerada

(This chapter draws on material previously published as: C. Gerada (2000) Drug Misuse and Primary Care in the New NHS. *Drugs: Education, Prevention and Policy*, 7(3): 213–223.)

Introduction

From the early 1980s onwards, central government policy in the UK has been to involve general practitioners (GPs) in the care of drug misusers (see, for example, the 1982 'Treatment and Rehabilitation' report from the Advisory Council on the Misuse of Drugs; and the 1984 'Orange Guidelines' from the Department of Health). High morbidity and mortality rates make it particularly important that drug misusers make contact with treatment services, though for well-rehearsed reasons this group is regularly denied effective and evidence-based treatment by the National Health Service (perhaps the only patients to whom this applies so blatantly).

To move forward, it is important for GPs to feel able to undertake the care of these patients and it is also important to ensure that mechanisms are in place to support and train these general practitioners. Finally it is important that payment structures reflect the increased work that caring for this group of patients brings.

This chapter describes, from an English primary care perspective, the changing face of primary care, its altered relationship to secondary care and how primary care can best act to provide a service to patients with substance-related problems. It also attempts to guide the reader through some of the key policy changes that have occurred that are relevant to planning and delivering a service to substance-misuse patients.

Primary care – present state

For most patients, primary care is the first point of contact with the health service. Ninety-eight per cent of the population is registered with a general practitioner (GP) and 60–70 per cent of this registered population will see their GP each year (Sharpe and Morrell, 1989). Collectively one to one and a half million patient contacts are made by about 30,000 GPs and around 20,000 primary care nurses every day, each contact lasting an average of 7.5 minutes (Goldberg, 1991). This makes the GP and the primary care nurse a vital component of any mental health and drug strategy and a useful early warning sign of developing health problems.

One of the most distinctive characteristics of primary care in the UK is that it is a readily accessible service, accessed by self-referral, to a registered population usually involving all members of a family, provided in a community setting by general practitioners and primary care nurses working with a wider health care team (Gerada, 2001).

Many countries have developed primary care services with variations in the structure and organisation, mode of payment of GPs, gatekeeper function and relationship to secondary specialist services. Where primary care is most developed, such as the Netherlands, Denmark, United Kingdom and Canada, the GP forms the core and focal point of the primary health care team. He or she is the first point of contact for most patients, including drug users, and provides generalist and increasingly specialist care to these patients. In these countries the GP provides personal care for individuals in the context of their families, their community and culture, and exercise their professional role by promoting health, preventing disease and providing cure, care and palliation (Horder, 1983).

Changing climate

Since the 1990s, primary care in the United Kingdom has undergone considerable change in organisation, services and payment structure. A plethora of new organisations and strategies have been launched in recent years – see Table 6.1. Change continues and from April 2004 general practitioners have been working under a new General Medical Service contract.

Beginning with the introduction of fund-holding and the purchaser– provider split of the early 1990s, these major changes continued with the 1997 NHS Primary Care Act and the changes in the organisation of primary care laid out in *The New NHS, Modern, Dependable* (Department of Health, 1997). The Primary Care Act heralded the ability of other professional groups such as nurses to provide primary care services, not necessarily through the traditional surgery environment. For example, through nurse-led Walk-in Clinics offering care to any patient and NHS Direct, a nurse-led telephone advice and information service. The most recent Government Plan, the NHS Plan (Department of Health, 2000) heralds new roles for nurses and general practitioners, in particular through the development of intermediate (general practitioners with special clinical interest) practitioners able to offer new

Table 6.1 Policy and other changes

New NHS, Modern and Dependable – formation of Primary Care Trusts putting
  greater emphasis on locally determined services and pooled budgets
NHS Plan – new roles for GPs, pharmacists and nurses
RCGP – accreditation of general practitioners with special clinical interest
New GP Contract – dividing GP work into core and enhanced categories with
  resource and payment implications
National Treatment Agency – co-ordinating services and improving quality and
  standards
Shipman Inquiry – possibly curtailing the range and amounts of controlled drugs that
  can be prescribed by general practitioners

Source: Author.

ways of providing services to their colleagues. Changes in regulations will also give much greater prescribing rights to nurses and pharmacists, these rights including controlled drugs. This chapter attempts to explain some of the major NHS policies and the changing climate of service delivery impacts on the care of drug users.

New organisations

The New NHS, Modern and Dependable – *Primary Care Groups and Primary Care Trusts*

The formation of Primary Care Groups and the development of Primary Care Trusts (NHS Executive, 1999) are a key part of the changes described in *The New NHS, Modern and Dependable.* Primary Care Groups (PCGs) became live in April 1999 and from April 2000 were superseded by Primary Care Trusts (PCTs). PCTs are free-standing, statutory bodies with new flexibilities and freedoms. They have their own budget for local health care and are able to develop new integrated services that combine social and health care. Like their forerunner PCGs, they have GPs at Board level (though in fewer numbers) and attempt to develop a 'bottom-up/top-down' approach to planning services that aim to make services reflect local needs. The functions of Primary Care Trusts are to improve the health of the community, develop primary care community health services and commission secondary care services.

Primary Care Trusts are the basic organisational framework for the delivery and organisation of all primary, community and increasingly social health care services. Each serves a population of around 100–250,000 patients, across defined geographical boundaries, usually coterminal with local authority boundaries. General practices and practitioners fall within these boundaries and collectively are expected to deliver services as defined by their Primary Care Trusts; these services in turn are determined by the needs laid out in national and locally determined service framework documents. In time, PCTs will influence more the location, organisation, staffing levels, and the types of services offered by and in primary care. In addition, it will be the responsibility of PCTs to ensure that all patients in their area are able to access effective health care, including treatment for substance misuse problems.

National Treatment Agency

A new National Treatment Agency (NTA) for England was established in April 2001. The NTA is expected to play a lead role in setting and monitoring drug treatment standards and to oversee a pooled national treatment budget.

New flexibilities

NHS Primary Care Act 1997

The 1997 NHS Primary Care Act was passed in the last few days of the Conservative Government and marked a revolutionary change in general practice. The launch of Personal Medical Services (PMS) pilot schemes effectively ended GPs' monopoly of primary medical care with new market entrants in the shape of Community Trusts and nurses. PMS services allowed general practitioners to define their own priorities determined on the needs of their local community. PMS pilots (pilots as each scheme was for a period of three years) were intended to give Health Authorities (HAs) (now Primary Care Trusts) and providers, particularly nurses, GPs and Community Trusts the flexibility and opportunity to innovate by offering different options for addressing primary care needs. GPs and nurses could now negotiate a salaried contract to provide services to meet local needs, such as refugees, homeless patients and drug users. PMS pilots proved very popular and provide a useful tool for the delivery of services to patients such as drug users who may find it hard to access primary care services. At the present time PMS services may be superseded by reforms heralded by the new GP contract, where theoretically GPs are able to define the level and type of service that their practice wishes to deliver. This will be discussed later in this chapter.

Example of Personal Medical Services (PMS) – Fulcrum Practice

In April 2001 the former Middlesbrough and Eston Primary Care Group set up its own Personal Medical Services pilot, the Fulcrum Medical Practice. This initiative, believed to be the first of its type in the UK, aimed to provide a 'first stop' service for people with addiction problems, enabling them to access general medical treatment and specialist help for their addiction problem. The Practice currently provides primary care and specialist drug dependency services to 500 patients. It works in partnership with other organisations with a remit of tackling drug misuse. Its aim is to engage more drug misusers, more quickly, into treatment and rehabilitation and to reduce the harmful effects of substance misuse on them, their families and the community.

In addition to the usual range of NHS Primary Care Services the practice offers specialist medical and nursing treatment of drug dependency. The practice also offers advice on the treatment of drug dependency to other general practitioners.

The NHS Plan

The NHS Plan is an ambitious but practical blueprint to modernise the NHS. It sets out the long-term plan for reform in the NHS, including the development of enhanced career opportunities for GPs (and nurses). The plan aims to create up to a thousand specialist GPs (in a range of different areas) who would be able to take referrals from fellow GPs.

The creation of the General Practitioner with Special Interest (GPwSI)

As discussed above, the NHS Plan has highlighted the need to create new careers for general practitioners – in particular to create 'Intermediate practitioners', stating 'that there will be a bigger role for general practitioners in shaping local services, as more become specialist GPs'. This initiative, perhaps led by a shortage of specialists and increasing hospital-waiting times, has been supported by the Royal College of General Practitioners (RCGP), who see it as a means of promoting portfolio careers and diversification amongst general practitioners (Royal College of General Practitioners, 2001). The College prefer the term General Practitioners with Special Interest (GPwSI) so as not to undermine the considerable expertise of the generalist practitioner.

The concept of the GPwSI is not new; many doctors have been working in this capacity for a number of years, largely unrecognised except within their local area. There are examples of GPs who are informally regarded as 'expert' within their own practice or immediate locality. What is new and both exciting and potentially threatening is that Primary Care Trusts can now commission these doctors to provide care outside the confines of the practice. Trusts will be able to, according to local need and expertise, define the number of practitioners, speciality areas, terms and conditions, pay and service-level agreements of these doctors. How these new roles develop and how they achieve the aims of reducing waiting times and provide fulfilling roles for GPs needs to be evaluated. Certainly, PCTs will need to understand and use the new expertise wisely so as to ensure that they are not merely replacing consultant specialist opinion with a cheaper, less experienced one.

Ideally the GPwSI should augment rather than replace specialist services, acting as an intermediate tier of expertise and advice to their primary care colleagues and at the same time provide an alternative avenue for referral. The Royal College of General Practitioners has developed a Certificate in Drug Misuse aimed at the GPwSI – an accredited qualification which took its first intake in 2001 (Gerada and Mumane, 2003). The first year saw approximately 400 GPs undertake the five-day training programme with around 80 per cent of the candidates successfully completing the requirements of the course.

The new GP contract (BMA, 2002)

The new GMS contract will bring about fundamental changes in GPs' terms and conditions of service, such that for the first time their payment structure will be more strictly defined and costed according to the type and quality of service they provide and according to patient experience of the service they receive. The contract will divide the general practitioners work into 'core', 'enhanced' and 'additional services'. Core services being acute self-limited illness or care of patients with terminal illness. Enhanced services will be those such as child health surveillance, chronic disease management, etc. Additional services, though as yet undefined, will undoubtedly include services such as those to drug users, the homeless and refugees. The new contract will also become a practice-based as opposed to practioner-based contract, and the implications of this still need to be explored.

The new contract should have opportunities for the development and provision of drug misuse treatment services. At best it will facilitate the development of local GP 'experts' or general practitioners with special clinical interest. As payment will be more closely matched to the type and level of care provided it would be possible for Primary Care Trusts to define service-level agreements and ensure that good quality care is maintained. Problems with the new contract may be that it will leave a few committed or maverick doctors looking after large numbers of drug users, hence returning to the unsatisfactory state of affairs of the 1980s. Nevertheless, the new contract gives more power to the PCT for defining, commissioning and funding services that best meet local needs. See Table 6.2 for a summary.

Table 6.2 Potential benefits of the new GP contract in relation to the care of drug users

Uniformity in payment structure
Uniformity of service-level agreements
Uniformity of standards of care
Care of drug users will be seen as more mainstream – rather than an 'optional extra' according to the whims of the locality
PCT will have a responsibility to ensure that services to drug users are provided

National policy, the GP and drug misuse

The World Health Organisation (WHO, 1973) as long ago as 1973, listed some of the crucial reasons why GPs are well placed to deliver primary care to those with mental illness, including drug and alcohol misuse, and many of these reasons have been discussed in Chapter 5, this volume. Policy makers have consistently prioritised the care of drug misusers by general practitioners and a number of policy documents, statements and key publications have been produced to this effect over the last decade.

RCGP/GPC joint statement

GPs' attitudes with regard to their role in the care of drug users has changed considerably over recent years. From a standpoint of 'leave to the specialist' there is now a definite belief that, given the right supports, training and resources, the GP has an important role to play. A joint policy statement, published in April 2000 by the two National Primary Care Bodies, reflects this shift in attitude and marked a watershed in primary care's involvement in the care of drug users:

> The RCGP and GPC believe that General Practitioners should offer appropriate care to all patients on their lists. Where patients have problems with substance abuse, appropriate care will include aspects of primary care normally provided by the practice health care team, shared care with other services and referral; to other appropriate services. Certain GPs may develop particular expertise in the care of substance abusers, and the number and location of these doctors should, ideally, be sufficient to avoid substantial workload falling onto only a few GPs. In supporting the development of this expertise, the Health Departments must ensure the provision of appropriate training in this field; facilitate professional support; resource the adequate provision for support services, including specialist service, and offer appropriate financial additional remuneration for such work.
>
> (RCGP/GPC Policy Statement on Care of
> Substance Abusers, 2000)

Drug strategy

The UK Government's 1998 White Paper 'Tackling Drugs to Build a Better Britain' set out to the Government's ten-year strategy for tackling drug misuse. It had four key themes: prevention, treatment, reducing availability and fighting drug-related crime. It emphasised the rights of drug misusers to receive treatment, including from primary care, and identified treatment in primary care as an important facet in delivery of this strategy. A key target was set – to increase participation of drug misusers in treatment by 66 per cent by 2005 and by 100 per cent by 2008.

Clinical guidelines (The Departments of Health, 1999)

The Department of Health published the new 'Guidelines on the Management of Drug Misuse and Dependence' (often referred to as the 'Orange Guidelines') in 1999 after a gap of nearly ten years. These set out the minimum responsibilities of the prescribing doctor and made some key recommendations, in particular:

- Responsibilities of all doctors to provide care to drug users for both general medical needs and for drug-related problems;
- Improved safety through good assessment procedures, urine analysis, dose assessment where possible, regular reviews and shared care working;
- Reducing diversion through daily dispensing and supervised ingestion;
- Provision of evidence-based interventions;
- Need to work within a shared care framework.

These new Guidelines emphasised the rights of drug users to receive appropriate care and stressed the responsibilities of all doctors to provide effective safe care. They offered a template for safe practice, in particular promoting shared care or collaborative working between different professional groups and between different levels of expertise.

Shared care

Shared care, or joint working, between the specialist and the generalist is seen as the ideal model to be used to facilitate primary care involvement. Shared care is defined as communication that goes beyond the simple exchange of a letter. No single model of shared care can be advocated; different arrangements must be developed depending on local drug service organisation, prevalence and type of drug use, availability of specialists and the organisation of primary care. A joint working group of the Royal College of Psychiatrists and GPs concluded that effective shared care could be achieved if some or all of the following measures were in place: close contact between GP and specialist; integrated training; audit; locally agreed management protocols;

and well-defined responsibility for control and monitoring of prescribing (Gerada and Farrell, 1998).

In the shared treatment of drug users the following are practical examples currently in operation.

* Consultant-led specialist service with full-time medical facilitator and nursing support (Greenwood, 1992). Patients assessed and stabilised at a clinic and then referred to participating GPs for opiate and benzodiazepine prescribing with a treatment plan that involves regular contact with a named key worker. Random urine testing and sanctions for continued illicit drug use. Changes in medication negotiated with community drug worker and case conferences called to address complications that arise. The specialist service manages only a small number of patients with complex needs.

* Staged care with consultant (psychiatrist or specialist GP or PAM practitioner allied to medicine) led drug team assessing and commencing treatment with central prescribing for an agreed limited period followed by GP taking over prescribing with support of a key worker attached to the practice or from specialist service. In some instances GP clinical assistants are involved in the assessments.

* Liaison team (led by consultant psychiatrist or general practioner with special clinical interest, or PAM) with a team of suitably qualified staff (alcohol and drug specialists) employed by specialist provider. The team is based in primary care and facilitates and supports GPs to manage the treatment of drug users. The team is peripatetic and aims to enable the GPs to treat the users rather than members of the team taking over care themselves (Gerada et al., 2000).

* A 'one-stop' clinic led by specialist general practitioner and employing a range of additional services, such as psychologist, social worker, drug and alcohol workers (Cohen and Schamroth, 1989). In some locations the GP sees referrals and carries out assessments on behalf of other GPs within a locality (Wilson et al., 1994). In this latter example, methadone maintenance clinics are run jointly by GPs and drug counsellors in two Glasgow practices. The patients are seen in separate clinics within general practice rather than during normal surgeries – which might otherwise inadvertently cause problems of stigmatisation and congregation of drug users. The GP is mainly involved in initial assessment of patients, stabilisation on methadone and then with inter-current illness and serological testing.

The way forward – towards an integrated local drug strategy

What follows is a practice example of how the policy initiatives can fit with other changes to bring about an effective drug and safe service. New models of services can now be developed and funded in a manner which is specifically designed to best meet local needs. Practitioners can be drawn from primary and secondary care, and include clinical leads from nursing and medical backgrounds. Perhaps the most exciting potential is how the new General Practitioner with Special Interest (GPwSI) can be used to best effect. Whatever the eventual way forward, it is important the Primary Care Trust involves all key stakeholders in the planning process and that all personnel are trained and supported at a level congruent with the service they are expected to provide.

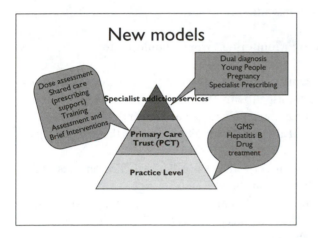

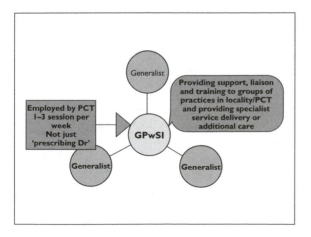

Figure 6.1 New models of care
Source: Author.

The following is an illustrative local action plan.

(Task 1) Establish a Shared Care Monitoring Group

The group ideally should include representation from

* Local medical committee
* Primary Care Trust
* Public health
* Lead drug and alcohol services (statutory and non-statutory)
* Drug action team representation

The role of Shared Care Monitoring Group should be to:

* Approve local payment agreements (it may be that National guidance will be established with the new GP contract; as yet no guidance exists and recommended rates vary depending on the roles and responsibilities of the GP undertaking care of the drug user);
* Clarify performance indicators;
* Monitor the delivery and effectiveness of shared care services and primary care involvement in the area;
* Take a strategic overview of shared care and primary care drug services and ensure that they keep abreast with new developments in treatment and rehabilitation.

(Task 2) Local Needs Assessment

* Establish the extent of the local drug problem;
* Establish types of drugs used in the locality and any special problems within the area;
* Identify current providers (specialist, general practitioner with special clinical interest (GPwSI), nurse consultant, generalist and voluntary (non-statutory) sector personnel);
* Identify key gaps in service providers;
* Identify potential providers;
* Review training needs and establish training strategy to meet these needs.

(Task 3) Establish local shared care guidelines

Locally agreed guidelines for the treatment of drug misusers, using National Guidelines as a framework, need to be drawn together and agreed. Guidelines should include:

- Standardised assessment treatment and referral guidelines. These might include standardised acceptance criteria, initial and on-going assessment, referral to specialist services, clear prescribing guidelines including minimum and maximum recommended doses, drug treatment regimes, frequency of prescribing criteria for review, etc.;
- Establish service-level agreement with those involved in shared care. Included in this would be guidelines on the minimum expected from the generalist and the GPwSI;
- Define the roles and responsibility of professionals participating in shared care. This should identify skills, knowledge and experience of the providers as well as the service specification. These definitions should be based on any national guidance, including that from the National Treatment Agency core competencies and the RCGP Certificate in Drug Misuse;
- Mechanisms for support for practitioners involved in the care of drug users;
- Monitoring and evolution mechanisms, including making payments (part or all) to measure performance such as notification to the Drug Misuse Regional DataBase.

Conclusion

The changes described in the new NHS mean that services should now be defined to meet needs, rather than the needs adapting to fit the service. Finally, the drug-dependent patient may be able to break out of the straight-jacket bed. In future, in addition to the wider provision of basic medical care to the drug misuser by the broad mass of GPs, the provision of more complicated assessments and treatments will be undertaken by the new generation of GPwSI – general practitioners who have a special interest and who receive ongoing further training to support their enhanced status and increased responsibilities. The new GPwSI will also act as a resource for their local colleagues. All these changes mean that primary care can, from now on, play a major and important role in the care of drug users.

References

Audit Commission (2002). Changing Habits. The commissioning and management of community drug treatment services for adults. Audit Commission Publications (www.audit-commission.gov.uk).

Cohen, J. and Schamroth, A. (1989). General practice management of drug misusers. *The Practitioner*, 233: 1471–1474.

Department of Health (2000). The NHS Plan. London: HMSO.

Drug Misuse and Dependence, Guidelines on Clinical Management (1999). Department of Health, The Scottish Office Department of Health, Welsh Office Department of Health and Social Services, Northern Ireland. London: The Stationery Office.

General Practitioners Committee (2002). Your contract, your future. BMA (www.bma.org.uk).

Gerada, C. (2001). Primary Care Service for Mental Health. In R. Ramsay, C. Gerada, S. Mars and G. Szmukler (eds) *Mental Illness. A Handbook for Carers*. London: Jessica Kingsley.

Gerada, C. and Farrell, M. (1998). Shared care. In R. Robertson (ed.) *Management of Drug Users in the Community: A Practical Handbook*. London: Arnold, 328–352.

Gerada, C. and Mumane, M. (2003). Royal College of General Practitioners Certificate in Drug Misuse. *Drugs: Education, Prevention and Policy*, 10(4): 369–379.

Gerada, C., Barrett, C., Betterton, J. and Tighe, J. (2000). The Consultancy Liaison Addiction Service – the first five years of an integrated, primary care based community drug and alcohol team. *Drugs: Education, Prevention and Policy*, 7: 251–256.

Goldberg, D. (1991). Filters to care – a model. In R. Jenkins and S. Griffiths (eds) *Indicators for Mental Health in the Population: A Series of Two Workshops*. London: HMSO.

Greenwood, J. (1992). Persuading general practitioners to prescribe – good husbandry or recipe for chaos? *British Journal of Addiction*, 87: 567–578.

Horder, J. (1983). General practice in 2000: Alma Ata Declaration. *British Medical Journal*, 286: 191–194.

NHS Primary Care Act (1997).

Primary Care Trusts: Establishing Better Services (1999). NHS Executive, April: 98C753/241.

Royal College of General Practitioners (2001). General Practitioners with Special Interests. London (www.rcgp.org.uk/recgp/corporate/responde/nhsplan/Gpspecialinterests).

Sharpe, D. and Morrell, D. (1989). The psychiatry of general practices. In P. Williams, G. Wilkinson and K. Rawnsely (eds) *The Scope of Epidemiological Psychiatry*. London: Routledge.

Tackling Drugs to Build a Better Britain: The Government's 10-Year Strategy for Tackling Drug Misuse (1998). London: The Stationery Office.

The New NHS: Modern, Dependable (1997). London: The Stationery Office.

WHO, Primary Care of Mental Illness (1973). Geneva.

Wilson, P., Watson, R. and Ralston, G. E. (1994). Methadone maintenance in general practice patients, workload and outcomes. *British Medical Journal*, 309: 641–644.

Chapter 7

Treating drug dependence in primary care

Reflecting on the problems as well as the potential

John Merrill and Sue Ruben

(This chapter is adapted from material originally published in journal form as: Merrill, J. and Ruben, S. (2000) Treating drug dependence in primary care: worthy ambition but flawed policy? *Drugs: Education, Prevention and Policy*, 7, 203–212.)

Introduction

UK national policy aims to increase the role of general practitioners in treating drug dependence. By working in 'shared care' arrangements with specialist services they will become the main providers of treatment and, in particular, of methadone maintenance. There is little evidence to support the effectiveness of this approach. Studies on GPs' attitudes to treating drug users, their knowledge and prescribing practices give rise to concern. Though examples of good practice by a minority of GPs are expanding, a national drug treatment policy should not be based on descriptive models of care alone. The foundations for an evidence-based policy must be substantiated.

Compared to other countries, the UK is unique in having minimal restrictions on how doctors treat drug dependence (Strang and Gossop, 1994). Such freedom allows any doctor to prescribe virtually any drug to their patients. The only legal controls limit prescribing heroin, cocaine and Diconal (dipipanone) to doctors who have obtained special licences from the Home Office. These restrictions were imposed as a result of injudicious and overly-generous prescribing of these drugs in the late 1960s. This marked a change in policy which encouraged the management of addiction by specialists in drug dependence. At the same time, those with little or no training or experience in managing drug misuse can, and do, prescribe injectable methadone, morphine and amphetamine to addicts.

The relative absence of rules and regulations that characterise the 'British System' allows prompt and flexible responses to the changing nature of drug problems (Strang and Gossop, 1994). The rapid and widespread adoption of syringe exchange schemes and the belated acceptance of methadone maintenance was thus facilitated. As a consequence HIV rates amongst British injecting drug users are extraordinarily low (Stimson, 1995). As the late 1980s saw a shift in emphasis in UK drugs policy towards public health, the late 1990s witnessed another shift in the predominant agenda to that of crime reduction. Having accepted that 'treatment works' the emphasis is now firmly on bringing more heroin users into treatment (Department of Health, The Scottish Office Department of Health, Welsh Office Department of Health and Social Services, Northern Ireland, 1999). However, some areas of the UK are bereft of specialist treatment services and many drug services are unable to meet the demand for treatment. The Government's solution is to encourage GPs to take a greater role in treating drug users and, in particular, to prescribe methadone maintenance for heroin dependence in 'shared care' arrangements with specialist services. This represents a distinct shift in policy. Over the last three decades GPs have been urged to treat medical complications of drug misuse and to provide detoxification by methadone reduction but not methadone maintenance (Department of Health, Scottish Office, Welsh Office, 1991).

Management of drug misuse in primary care: what is the evidence base?

There is a paucity of evidence to support the management of drug misuse by GPs. Several papers have reported outcomes on the management of heroin dependence in general practice, but treatments have varied considerably and outcomes have been inconsistent and ill-defined (Cohen et al., 1992; Martin et al., 1998; Peters and Reid, 1998; Ford and Ryrie, 1999; Gossop et al., 1999). In contrast, attitudes of GPs to treating drug misuse (Glanz, 1986; Abed and Neira-Munoz, 1990; Bell, 1990; Davies and Huxley, 1997; Deehan et al., 1997) and opinions of drug users on being treated by their GPs (Bennett and Wright, 1986; McKeganey, 1988; Telfer and Clulow, 1990; Gerada et al., 1992; Hindler et al., 1996) have received considerable attention and produced more consistent results.

Outcomes

Cohen et al. (1992) described treatment of 150 heroin users in a central London general practice. Methadone maintenance was not offered, only detoxification. At three-month follow-up, half were reported to be drug free, but 21 patients were undergoing residential detoxification and in 23 cases no urinalysis was available to substantiate self-reports of abstinence. Wilson et al. (1994) evaluated the outcome of methadone maintenance prescribed for 46 injecting heroin users in Glasgow. They found no evidence of illicit opiate use (based on self-report or urinalysis) in the week preceding 78 per cent of patients' consultations. Only four patients elected to have a methadone detoxification and all failed to achieve abstinence.

Less impressive outcomes were reported on a much larger group of 494 heroin users treated at the Edinburgh service (Peters and Reid, 1998). Treatment retention over 12 months was only 39 per cent. Significant reductions in both injecting and criminal behaviour were achieved but there was no improvement in sharing injecting equipment, use of condoms, illicit drug use or employment. Unfortunately the study was marred by over-simplistic questioning about illicit drug use at follow-up which may have resulted in an under-estimation of the benefits of treatment.

The only study comparing treatment outcomes in general practice and at specialist services was drawn from a sample of the National Treatment Outcome Research Study (NTORS) (Gossop *et al.*, 1999). At six-month follow-up, similar improvements were obtained in 155 patients receiving 'methadone treatment' within general practice and 297 treated at specialist services. Methadone treatment included those prescribed reducing and maintenance doses. The number of patients receiving reducing or maintenance treatment was not specified, nor was any indication given as to how many completed detoxification. Frequency of heroin use fell to less than half that at intake with significant reductions in the use of other drugs but not alcohol. However, as the authors emphasise, these results cannot be generalised as the seven general practices involved were atypical, including five that co-ordinated shared care for 35 other practices and two that provided treatment for large numbers of drug users.

There is a pressing need for randomised controlled studies comparing the outcome of treating drug users within specialist services and through shared care with GPs. As yet, the evidence base for the effectiveness of treatment within general practice is sorely lacking.

Prescribing practice

Evidence derived from a national study of community pharmacies indicates poor GP prescribing practices (Strang *et al.*, 1996). Although GPs write over 40 per cent of prescriptions for methadone, they are less likely than specialist services to prescribe methadone in the form of methadone mixture and for daily dispensing. Prescribing amphetamine is recognised as being very much within the specialist remit but 43 per cent of dexamphetamine prescriptions were issued by GPs (Strang and Sheridan, 1997). A follow-up study examining changes in prescribing practices as a result of recommendations for doctors to prescribe methadone in the form of mixture rather than tablets and for more frequent dispensing yielded worrying results (Strang and Sheridan, 1998). This demonstrated a 20 per cent increase in prescribing methadone but no significant change towards prescribing mixture or daily dispensing. The authors concluded, 'If planners are awaiting major change in methadone prescribing as a result of exhortation, they should not hold their breath.'

Inconsistencies in GP prescribing can be further illustrated by comparing the methadone detoxification-only policy described by Cohen *et al.* above with that reported in two other reports. Martin and colleagues (Martin *et al.*, 1998), working in Bedford with no specialist service support, prescribed injectable methadone to 37 per cent of their heroin-dependent patients. Ford and Ryrie (1999) described prescribing injectable methadone by three GPs. One-quarter of those receiving methadone were prescribed the injectable form and nearly one-third were also prescribed dexamphetamine. Alarmingly, 34 per cent did not have urine samples analysed before injectable prescribing was initiated and only 30 per cent were notified to the regional drug misuse database. Perhaps not surprisingly in view of this relatively liberal practice patients 'rate their current treatment more favourably than previous specialist treatment'. Successive clinical guidelines on the management of drug dependence have viewed prescribing injectable drugs and dexamphetamine as being unproven treatments suitable only for a small minority of patients in specialist treatment (Department of Health, The Scottish Office Department of Health, Welsh Office Department of Health and Social Services, Northern Ireland, 1999).

In summary, these reports indicate GPs have not responded to previous advice and guidelines on responsible and safe prescribing practices.

Attitudes to treating drug misuse in general practice

There has been an abundance of research on attitudes of GPs towards treating drug misuse which demonstrates consistent results. A study of a 5 per cent sample of GPs in England and Wales found 76 per cent believed that opiate users presented more severe management problems than any other group of patients (Glanz, 1986). Only 23 per cent felt they were competent to treat drug users but 45 per cent stated they would be more willing to be involved if back-up services were available. Those who qualified more recently had less unfavourable attitudes. Similarly only 16 per cent of London GPs felt they had adequate training to manage opiate dependence and 35 per cent stated they would be more willing to treat drug misusers if they had further training (Bell, 1990). In Norwich the vast majority of GPs did not consider drug addiction to be a medical problem and 76 per cent felt the management of drug misuse was beyond their competence (Abed and Neira-Munoz, 1990). Very few believed there was any role for prescribing in primary care. If indicated, they thought it should be provided by a specialist service.

More recent studies have shown similar results in other parts of the country. Although 80 per cent of GPs in Greater Manchester prescribed for drug users only 20 per cent felt sure that treatment was within the competence of GPs. Sixty-one per cent believed they lacked the necessary knowledge to prescribe, and most had not read the Department of Health's Guidelines on Clinical Management, distributed free to all doctors (Davies and Huxley,

1997). Although 60 per cent believed that shared care provided the best treatment, only 20 per cent disagreed with the statement that all opiate users should be referred on to specialist services. Most believed that more training would encourage GP treatment but such sentiments were not found in London where the majority of GPs believed drug users should not be treated in primary care, and that neither additional training nor financial inducements would significantly change their attitudes (Deehan et al., 1997).

Reciprocating the generally negative attitudes of GPs towards treating drug users are those of drug users towards treatment by GPs. Only a quarter of drug users attending a specialist clinic had ever consulted their GPs for a drug-related matter although their mean duration of dependence was over four years (Telfer and Clulow, 1990). Reasons for not disclosing drug misuse to GPs include finding GPs lacking in knowledge and understanding, being critical and unsympathetic (Bennett and Wright, 1986; Telfer and Clulow, 1990; Hindler et al., 1996) and finding GPs unable to offer a treatment plan (McKeganey, 1988).

Thus there is considerable evidence to show that GPs are reluctant to prescribe for drug users. The lack of training, knowledge and experience of GPs in managing drug misuse is pertinent both to why GPs are averse to prescribing, and why drug users are disinclined to seek treatment from their GPs.

Assumed benefits of managing drug misuse within general practice

The assumed benefits of providing treatment within general practice include earlier intervention, greater knowledge of the drug user and their family, better treatment of physical health problems, patient preference for GP treatment and cost-effectiveness.

That drug use is no longer marginal but is commonplace amongst large sections of society and that early brief advice from GPs has been shown to be beneficial for nicotine and alcohol dependence are, for Carnwath et al. (2000), reasons why it is essential that GPs become more involved in treating drug dependence. Whilst the benefit of GPs gaining more knowledge of drug misuse is unquestionable, the overwhelming majority of those patients who use drugs are occasional cannabis smokers and do not require treatment at all. It seems unlikely that many dependent heroin users would stop using after receiving simple advice from a GP or any other professional. The value of 'brief interventions' for opiate dependence in a manner analogous to alcohol and nicotine has not been evaluated.

Gerada (2000) places much value on the role of GPs as family doctors, having continuing contact with patients and their families over many years, that 97 per cent of the population is registered with a GP and that drug users prefer to be treated by their GPs. However, considerable research demontrates that drug users are more likely to remain unregistered with GPs (only 38 per cent registered in Gerada's own research), to have been registered with their current GP for only a short period, to conceal their drug problem from their GP, and to prefer treatment by specialist services (Bennett and Wright, 1986; McKeganey, 1988; Gerada *et al.*, 1992; Telfer and Clulow, 1990). Hindler and colleagues studied drug users attending a community drug team, a drug dependence unit, a private clinic, a street agency and a general practice specialising in treating drug users (Hindler *et al.*, 1996). They found that most drug users sought out a GP who was prepared to treat them rather than register with a local or their family doctor. Most felt their GPs held negative views about them. Only the subgroup of 35 patients treated by the GPs with a special interest believed their doctors had a positive view of drug users.

A further assumption is that GPs are best placed to treat physical consequences of drug misuse. This would seem to be obvious even for those receiving treatment for drug dependence at specialist services. However, a report on Wirral Drug Service, a very large primary care-led service, found drug users were reluctant to attend their GPs for physical problems, even if their GP prescribes them methadone (Speed and Janikiewicz, 2000). They have developed a physical assessment and drop-in clinic for physical problems based within their specialist service and cite evidence that this is more cost-effective than relying on patients' own GPs to provide such services.

The cost of treating drug dependence in general practice is often assumed to be cheaper than specialist services but with little justification. Providing methadone maintenance in Glasgow was costed at £2,030 per patient annually in the early 1990s (Wilson *et al.*, 1994). This was based on an average of 20 minutes weekly of counsellor time and 3 minutes weekly of GP time and included the cost of methadone and chemists' dispensing fees. Costings are not available for comparison with specialist treatment but it would seem unlikely that specialist service cost would be higher and they may be much cheaper because staff costs would be similar but specialist services are likely to have more streamlined systems operating. As Lawrence (2000) notes, single-site drug services are likely to be less expensive than those split across sites, e.g. through shared care. The time spent travelling between sites can be substantial and shared care in other specialities has been shown not to be cost-effective (Black *et al.*, 1997). Further, the cost of training and supporting GPs is likely to be high.

In summary, the assumed benefits of providing treatment within general practice are not supported by research evidence.

Models of treatment by GPs

There is no recommended framework in which GPs work with drug users. Models of care have evolved taking into consideration geography, available expertise, prevalence and services already provided (Gerada and Tighe, 1999).

Five recent papers describe different models for providing treatment for drug dependence within general practice.

The Edinburgh model (Watson, 2000) began in 1988 and is the original and most influential shared care service for treating opiate dependence. The central specialist service provides assessment and treatment recommendations for GPs who are supported by staff from the specialist service. The rapid spread of HIV amongst injecting drug users in Edinburgh was undoubtedly a powerful motivating factor for GPs to prescribe. Seventy per cent of practices participate in the scheme. Watson's account provides a fascinating description of the natural history of the oldest shared care scheme in the UK that should prepare more recent schemes for what they can expect in the future. Support for GPs beyond the assistance of drug workers (in the form of a Primary Care Facilitation Team) was needed. GPs became disenchanted because many patients continued to use heroin and few moved towards abstinence. Many began to set quotas of patients they would treat, necessitating the establishing of 'locality clinics' to treat those who had exceeded the capacity of primary care. Ultimately the GPs expressed high levels of satisfaction with the Community Drug Problem Service, but the majority believed that prescribing should be left to the specialist service and 43 per cent had adopted a policy not to prescribe in the future.

Carnwath *et al.* (2000) describe primary care treatment for drug misusers in Greater Manchester with particular reference to Trafford. The Trafford service provides shared care in a similar manner to Edinburgh with the exception that treatment is initiated by GPs with the support of drug liaison workers. Interestingly the authors consider the question as to whether patients receive better treatment for their drug misuse in shared care or from specialist services as of secondary importance. Their primary aim is to encourage GPs to provide better general health care to drug users. Nevertheless, Trafford is probably unique in having encouraged all local GPs to prescribe methadone. How this considerable feat has been achieved is described in detail with reference to five stages of GP involvement. Why Trafford consider increasing the proportion of GPs prescribing from 60 per cent to 90 per cent as 'usually reasonably easy' when Edinburgh and other areas of Greater Manchester have plateaued at 70–80 per cent (Watson, 2000; Davies and Huxley, 1997) is not clear. Circulating publications demonstrating the effectiveness of methadone maintenance is thought to be helpful but perhaps unlikely to convince the more perceptive GPs who may recognise all of this is based on treatment at specialist services. Trafford is distinct from other areas in Greater Manchester in encompassing some affluent areas, and having particularly good GPs. It also has a high quality, 'evangelistic' drug service which has been successful in attracting considerable funds for expanding shared care.

In London, the Consultancy Liaison Addiction Service (CLAS) described by Gerada *et al.* (2000) introduces an intermediate tier between specialist services and GPs. With only five full-time staff, CLAS undertakes extensive training and treatment remits for both alcohol and drug misuse. These functions would usually be undertaken by the specialist service working in a shared care paradigm. Unfortunately no indication is given as to the extent of involvement with, or the treatments offered to, the 928 drug misusers seen by the service. CLAS concentrates their efforts on those practices most willing to work with substance misusers and this begs the question as to what happens to those patients who are registered with the remaining GPs? This problem could be addressed by Gerada et al.'s innovative idea of encouraging the more committed GPs to become specialised generalists and act as expert resources for their more reticent colleagues.

The Wirral Drug Service (Speed and Janikiewicz, 2000) is unusual in being a large specialist drug service that is led by a GP. A similar large GP-led specialist service exists in Glasgow (Gruer et al., 1997). The Wirral service comprises a core substitute prescribing service and branches of the service dealing specifically with outreach, physical healthcare, mental health, young drug users, female and pregnant drug users, and GP liaison. Wirral Drug Service differs markedly from Trafford in providing extensive facilities that would normally be expected to be provided by patients' own GPs. These include a 'drop-in' clinic for physical problems, physical health assessment, cervical smears and contraception. Despite a core component of the service being to reintegrate patients into primary care, they have been less successful in achieving this aim than the specialist psychiatry-led drug services in Greater Manchester. Fewer than one-third of their patients are prescribed for by their own GPs and the service's GP liaison workers work with only a minority of general practices.

Lawrence (2000) describes the management of drug misuse almost exclusively within a general practice in the Chapletown area of Leeds. The GPs along with an addiction counsellor provide a high level of expertise. Indeed they are funded by the health authority to provide a secondary level (specialist) service to their patients. The paper acknowledges the GPs' unusually high commitment to providing addiction services and makes no pretence that their model can be adopted universally. The authors are frank about the service's limitations in comparison to most specialist services and balance these deficits with the advantages of treatment provision wholly within general practice. Unusually for a specialist service, less than 10 per cent of their clients are offered long-term maintenance. Only two referrals were made to the well-developed specialist service at Leeds Addiction Unit.

These five recent descriptions of treating drug misuse within general practice demonstrate a range of models. In all five, treatment of the majority of drug users is carried out by GPs with support from experienced drug workers. Three are clearly specialist services – two (Edinburgh and Trafford) led by consultant psychiatrists specialising in drug misuse and one (Wirral) led by a GP. All three encourage treatment within shared care arrangements though Trafford has been much more successful in achieving this aim than Wirral, and in Edinburgh initial success has been followed by evidence of GP disillusion. Two are quasi-specialist services. CLAS is led by a specialised generalist who trained both in psychiatry and drug dependence and provides an intermediate tier between general practice and specialist services. In Chapletown the GPs are not specialists, work almost entirely independently from the local specialist services but receive funding for providing specialist treatment. CLAS acts as a specialist service in supporting shared care with GPs. In Chapletown shared care is eschewed.

A general practice-based drug treatment policy: problems with implementation in the UK

Will GPs do it?

For the Government's policy to work there will have to be a substantial change of attitude by GPs. An olive branch is seen in those studies that show younger GPs have less negative views and that many GPs believe further training and support will encourage them to treat more drug users. However, younger GPs have probably always been more enthusiastic about most aspects of their work, becoming less so as they age. Further training and support is not wanted by a considerable proportion of GPs (Deehan et al., 1997). Also, some of those that say more training would encourage them to treat drug users may not actually take up training opportunities, or may not subsequently treat more drug-using patients. Sadly, the baseline from which GPs have to be trained may have fallen as the amount of time devoted to training British medical students in substance misuse declined to half between 1987 and 1996 (Crome, 1999).

GPs do not only have to become more amenable to treating drug misusers, but they must also continue to treat them. In Edinburgh GPs are reluctant to accept the concept of the duration of methadone maintenance being unlimited and are tiring of treating drug users who may show little motivation towards abstinence (Watson, 2000).

Running counter to the UK Government's desire to increase GPs' involvement in the management of drug misuse, the doctor's representative body, the British Medical Association, specifically excluded methadone maintenance from its definition of core 'general medical services' that should be provided by GPs. Thus the BMA viewed methadone maintenance as an optional activity for GPs which, if provided, should attract extra payment (General Medical Services Committee, 1996).

Will GPs do it well?

In addition to 'will GPs do it?' the question 'will they do it well?' is crucial. The benchmark for quality of treatment will be the recent Clinical Guidelines

(Department of Health, The Scottish Office Department of Health, Welsh Office Department of Health and Social Services, Northern Ireland, 1999). These set more exacting guidelines than previous editions and carry a warning of legal liability if they are not followed. This may prove to further deter GP involvement. Standards of GP treatment will be regulated by local shared care monitoring groups. How these groups will operate when shared care remains loosely defined and is applicable in different guises from one general practice to another is uncertain. Similarly unclear is whether monitoring groups will have sanctions available for cases of poor practice or whether they will be in essence toothless.

What will it cost?

Training and supporting GPs will be expensive. Recently, these costs have been offset by subsidies from health authorities, 'top slicing' from GP budgets and funding through non-health sources such as urban regeneration budgets. An anomaly whereby health authorities have much of the cost of methadone prescribing by GPs (but not specialist services) paid from central NHS funds is about to end. Primary Care Trusts will not be subjected to compulsory top-slicing and non-health sources are likely to be reluctant to fund schemes which are no longer innovatory but are mainstream policy. The costs of training and support and the costs of monitoring shared care have not been evaluated.

What about specialist services?

Specialist services are essential for training and supporting GPs and managing chaotic drug users, those with multiple dependencies and co-morbid psychiatric disorders (Farrell and Gerada, 1997; Department of Health, The Scottish Office Department of Health, Welsh Office Department of Health and Social Services, Northern Ireland, 1999; Gerada, 2000). The UK has a shortage of specialist drug dependence doctors. By diverting resources towards cajoling often-reluctant GPs into treating drug users there is a danger that specialising in drug misuse may become an even less attractive career option.

Finally, the effect of fully implementing a primary-care-led NHS with Primary Care Groups giving GPs a leading role in determining local health service priorities and funding is uncertain. PCGs may decide to commission specialist services to treat their patients and thus be able to ignore national guidance. This may result in an even more confused and uncoordinated approach than is currently the case.

It is likely that the British System will endure because of unclear definitions about shared care, unworkable central guidance and, above all, too little evidence on which to base service commissioning. Having embarked

upon a national policy without a firm evidence base, the UK Government's Department of Health may be reluctant to fund research that could undermine their policy. Research on the effectiveness of treating drug users within general practice may, like the most renowned example of the British System – heroin prescribing – ultimately have to be provided from overseas.

References

Abed, R. and Neira-Munoz, E. (1990). A survey of general practitioners' opinion and attitude to drug addicts and addiction. *British Journal of Addiction*, 85, 131–136.

Bell, G. (1990). How willing are general practitioners to manage narcotic misuse? *Health Trends*, 22, 56–57.

Bennett, T. and Wright, R. (1986). Opioid users: attitudes towards the use of NHS clinics, general practitioners and private doctors. *British Journal of Addiction*, 81, 757–763.

Black, M., Leese, B., Gosden, T. and Mead, N. (1997). Specialist outreach clinics in general practice: what do they offer? *British Journal of General Practice*, 47, 558–561.

Carnwath, T., Gabbay, M. and Barnard, J. (2000). A share of the action: general practitioner involvement in drug misuse treatment in Greater Manchester. *Drugs: Education, Prevention and Policy*, 7, 235–250.

Cohen, J., Schamroth, A., Nazareth, I., Johnson, M., Graham, S. and Thomson, D. (1992). Problem drug use in a central London general practice. *British Medical Journal*, 304, 1158–1160.

Crome, I. B. (1999). The trouble with training: substance misuse education in British medical schools revisited. What are the issues? *Drugs: Education, Prevention and Policy*, 6, 111–123.

Davies, A. and Huxley, P. (1997). Survey of general practitioners' opinions on treatment of opiate users. *British Medical Journal*, 314, 1173–1174.

Deehan, A., Taylor, C. and Strang, J. (1997). The general practitioner, the drug misuser, and the alcohol misuser; major differences in general practitioner activity therapeutic commitment, and 'shared care' proposals. *British Journal of General Practice*, 47, 705–709.

Department of Health, Scottish Office, Welsh Office (1991). *Drug Misuse and Dependence. Guidelines on Clinical Management.* London, HMSO.

Department of Health, The Scottish Office Department of Health, Welsh Office, Department of Health and Social Services, Northern Ireland (1999). *Drug Misuse and Dependence – Guidelines on Clinical Management.* London: The Stationery Office.

Farrell, M. and Gerada, C. (1997). Drug misusers: whose business is it? *British Medical Journal*, 315, 559–560.

Ford, C. and Ryrie, I. (1999). Prescribing injectable methadone in general practice. *International Journal of Drug Policy*, 10, 39–45.

General Medical Services Committee (1996). *Core Services: Taking the Initiative.* London: British Medical Association.

Gerada, C. (2000). Drug misuse and primary care in the new NHS. *Drugs: Education, Prevention and Policy*, 7, 213–221.

Gerada, C. and Tighe, J. (1999). A review of shared care protocols for the treatment of problem drug use in England, Scotland and Wales. *British Journal of General Practice*, 439, 125–126.

Gerada, C., Orgel, M. and Strang, J. (1992). Health clinics for problem drug users. *Health Trends*, 24, 68–69.

Gerada, C., Barrett, C., Betterton, C. and Tighe, J. (2000). The Consultancy Liaison Addiction Service – the first five years of an integrated primary care-based community drug and alcohol team. Anonymous. *Drugs: Education, Prevention and Policy*, 7, 251–256.

Glanz, A. (1986). Findings of a national survey of the role of general practitioners in the treatment of opiate misuse: views on treatment. *British Medical Journal*, 293, 543–545.

Gossop, M., Marsden, J., Stewart, D., Lehmann, P. and Strang, J. (1999). Methadone treatment practices and outcome for opiate addicts treated in drug clinics and in general practice: results from the National Treatment Outcome Research Study. *British Journal of General Practice*, 49, 31–34.

Gruer, L., Wilson, P., Scott, R., Elliott, L., Macleod, J., Harden, K., Forrester, E., Hinshelwood, S., McNulty, H. and Silk, P. (1997). General practitioner centred scheme for treatment of opiate dependent drug injectors in Glasgow. *British Medical Journal*, 314, 1730–1735.

Hindler, C., King, M., Nazareth, I., Cohen, J., Farmer, R. and Gerada, C. (1996). Characteristics of drug misusers and their perceptions of general practitioner care. *British Journal of General Practice*, 46, 149–152.

Lawrence, S. (2000). Models of primary care for substance misusers: St Martins Practice, Chapletown, Leeds – secondary provision in a primary care setting. *Drugs: Education, Prevention and Policy*, 7, 279–291.

Martin, E., Canavan, A. and Butler, R. (1998). A decade of caring for drug users entirely within general practice. *British Journal of General Practice*, 48, 1679–1682.

McKeganey, N. (1988). Shadowland: general practitioners and the treatment of opiate-abusing patients in the UK. *British Journal of Addiction*, 83, 373–386.

Peters, A. D. and Reid, M. M. (1998). Methadone treatment in the Scottish context: outcomes of a community-based service for drug users in Lothian. *Drug and Alcohol Dependence*, 50, 47–55.

Speed, S. and Janikiewicz, S. M. J. (2000). Providing care to drug users on Wirral: a case study analysis of a Primary Health Care/General Practice-led service. *Drugs: Education, Prevention and Policy*, 7, 257–277.

Stimson, G. (1995). AIDS and injecting drug use in the United Kingdom, 1987–1993: the policy response and the prevention of the epidemic. *Social Science and Medicine*, 41, 699–716.

Strang, J. and Gossop, M. (1994). The 'British System': visionary anticipation or masterly inactivity? In *Heroin Addiction and Drug Policy*, edited by J. Strang and M. Gossop, Oxford: Oxford University Press.

Strang, J. and Sheridan, J. (1997). Prescribing amphetamines to drug misusers: data from the 1995 national survey of community pharmacies. *Addiction*, 92, 833–838.

Strang, J. and Sheridan, J. (1998). Effect of government recommendations on methadone prescribing in south east England: comparison of 1995 and 1997 surveys. *British Medical Journal*, 317, 1489–1490.

Strang, J., Sheridan, J. and Barber, N. (1996). Prescribing injectable and oral methadone to opiate addicts: results from the 1995 national postal survey of community pharmacies in England and Wales. *British Medical Journal*, 313, 270–272.

Telfer, I. and Clulow, C. (1990). Heroin misusers: what they think of their general practitioners. *British Journal of Addiction*, 85, 137–140.

Watson, F. (2000). Models of primary care for substance misusers: the Lothian experience. *Drugs: Education, Prevention and Policy*, 7, 223–234.

Wilson, P., Watson, R. and Ralston, G. E. (1994). Methadone maintenance in general practice: patients, workload, and outcomes. *British Medical Journal*, 309, 641–644.

Chapter 8

The rise and fall of the Community Drug Team

The gap between aspiration and achievement

Sue Clement and John Strang

(This chapter draws on material previously written by the authors and published in J. Strang and M. Gossop (eds) *Heroin Addiction and Drug Policy: The British System*, Oxford University Press, 1994.)

The introduction of Community Drug Teams (CDTs) in many parts of the UK was one of the major organizational changes to UK drug treatment services through the 1980s and 1990s. For the first time, instead of investing in specialist treatment units significant resources were targeted at the development of community-based services. Following the appointment of staff for the first CDT in 1983, there was a rapid expansion in the number of CDTs throughout the 1980s. By 1987, there were already 62 CDTs and by 1990 the number had grown to 75 (MacGregor *et al*. 1991). By 1991, a CDT had been established within more than half the 192 District Health Authorities in the country.

The end of an era?

The introduction of CDTs across the country went hand-in-hand with a fundamental shift in planning strategy in which it was envisaged that much of the care provided to drug users would be provided from within the mainstream of care delivery. The blueprint was contained within the Treatment and Rehabilitation Report from the Advisory Council on the Misuse of Drugs (ACMD 1982) which was heavily influenced by work done several years previously in the alcohol field (Maudsley Alcohol Pilot Project 1975; Shaw *et al*. 1978; Advisory Committee on Alcoholism 1978). The 1975 report by the Maudsley Alcohol Pilot Project had already outlined an approach in which the Community Alcohol Team (CAT) 'mobilised and integrated the potential skills of a variety of services, generic and specialist, at both primary and secondary levels'. This enabling role of the community team, with its emphasis on providing training and support to generic workers, rather than direct service provision, was in sharp contrast to what had gone before.

The new strategy was seen as heralding the end of an era with the death of the exclusive and excluding specialist. No longer was the problem of drug misuse to be seen as one for which a referral to the specialist was the only appropriate action. CDTs were to be the agents for the mobilization of generic services so that the management of drug misusers became but one additional client group in the rich tapestry of casework which forms the work of the generalist. It was a move from the specialist model to an integrated model of care delivery, in which the avenue of referral had become a two-way street (Strang 1989, 1991). It was a brave policy initiative but there proved to be many organizational barriers to its implementation.

The intended role of the CDT

Looking back on the policy guidance that was provided at the time for the development and running of a variety of community teams (mental health, mental handicap, alcohol, drugs, elderly) in the 1970s and 1980s, it is clear that the guidance lacked specificity. Hence it is unlike the emphasis which has been placed more recently on 'fidelity to the model' in the development of the new mental health services exemplified in Policy Implementation Guide (2001a). The reality of the 1980s and 1990s was that under the rubric of the 'community drug team' were gathered together a hotchpotch of different types of service, with much variation in size, disciplinary and skills mix, population served, etc., so that it was far from clear what were the common qualities of these various community teams.

Many of the CDTs established found themselves involved in having to try to work it out for themselves – attempting to work out the nature of their contribution as well as actually doing it. Despite the broad brush strokes available in the policy documents (for example, ACMD 1982) there was little detail provided by central government or local planners as to the precise operation of the services.

A number of factors have been identified as influencing the structure and aims of the early Community Drug Teams (Strang and Clement 1994):

(1)   The amount and nature of existing service provision – in areas with little or no specialist drug mis-use services – there were understandable pressures for CDTs to become directly involved in client care.

(2)   The available resources in the real world – the strategy adopted was influenced by the number and experience of full-time staff, and the extent to which sessional workers were seconded to the community service from generic services.

(3)   The locally identified needs of both clients and agencies – how the constituency of concern became defined and the criteria of 'caseness' adopted. Thus some CDTs went for a broad constituency (for example, see Schneider *et al.* 1989) whilst others presented a rationale for concentration

of resources on drug users who had already injected or might inject in the near future.

(4) The priority attached to multi-disciplinary team development – in the 1980s there was little detailed guidance about joint working mechanisms between health and social services and co-ordination was geographically variable as was the extent of non-statutory sector involvement in planning.

(5) Philosophy and professional background of service innovators – because little central guidance was given on the detailed working of teams, their development was sometimes part of an orchestrated expansion of services (for example, the network of CDTs in every district in the North Western Region (Strang et al. 1991)) whilst elsewhere the development was more parochial and was influenced almost exclusively by the attitudes and inclinations of local groups of workers (for example, see Schneider et al. 1989).

One common characteristic of all CDTs was their clear geographical brief – the CDT served defined populations. Thus all CDTs had a clear understanding of a people whom they served and of a geographical plot which was their responsibility. From this standpoint they were thought to be well positioned to be able to consider possible areas of unmet need to which services might be more specifically targeted – either geographical areas in which there was poor service access or uptake, or groups within the population who appeared not to be using the services for which they would appear to have a need. ACMD (1982) saw the CDT as playing a valuable role in local service planning.

The CDT model placed a heavy emphasis on working through and with primary care workers (ACMD 1982). However, it became clear over the next decade that the extent to which general practitioners (GPs) and other non-specialists were willing to become involved in the treatment of drug users made this problematic (Strang et al. 1991; Tantam et al. 1993). In some districts surveyed more than 90 per cent of local GPs were unwilling to be involved to any substantial extent with drug users (see Chapter 7, this volume).

The original blueprint for the CDT in the 1982 ACMD report regarded prescribing as but a small part of the broader response. However, there was early widespread evidence that the dominant activity and area of influence of the CDT worker had become the provision or non-provision of substitute drugs to the opiate addict. The substantial growth in the number of drug users on methadone maintenance programmes led to an increased demand for specialist services in the 1990s which led to the narrowing of the remit of CDTs even further. Whereas in the early 1980s most voluntary sector provision was concentrated on residential service provision, the subsequent growth in non-statutory counselling and outreach services in the 1990s further impacted on the function of CDTs. Increasingly non-statutory community services became relied upon to provide services such as counselling, with a medical model of management becoming dominant within the CDT.

Provision of advice, support and training to generic/non-specialist workers

The architects of community teams foresaw the impracticality of trying to offer a specialist service to everybody with drug- or alcohol-related problems; the number would be just too large for any specialist service to handle, nor was specialist intervention always required (Advisory Committee on Alcoholism 1978; ACMD 1982). In their original report, the Maudsley Alcohol Pilot Project (1975) identified three major factors underlying what was perceived as being the inadequate response of primary care worker to clients with alcohol problems:

(1)   anxieties about role adequacy (that is, not having the information and skills necessary to recognize and respond to the relevant cases);

(2)   anxieties about role legitimacy (that is, uncertainty as to the extent to which drinking problems formed a proper part of their professional responsibilities); and

(3)   anxieties about role support (the fear that there would be nowhere from which to obtain help and advice when they were unsure how or whether to respond).

These three factors conspired to create 'role insecurity', which led to 'low therapeutic commitment'. The obvious response was seen to be the provision of training in the areas of identification and responding to alcohol and drug problems to enable generic workers to take on this work. However, an early study identified that the provision of clinical information and training in counselling alone had no impact on the persistence of role insecurity. It was only when role support was added that the development of therapeutic commitment was facilitated (Cartwright 1980). Clement (1987) has further argued that the support of generic workers' line managers is a crucial factor in determining whether the worker sees intervention into alcohol or drug problems as being appropriate and indeed in determining whether participating in training is seen as a priority area.

In the drug field the responsibility for provision of the training of generic workers was placed largely with the newly emergent Regional Drug Training Units, established in several regions during the 1980s (Cranfield and Dixon 1990; Glass and Strang 1991). However, in reality the main recipients of training from these Regional Training Units were the newly created drug workers themselves. GPs were scarcely reached at all – for example, forming less than 2 per cent of the workers attending courses or seminars run by one such Regional Drug Training Unit (RDTU) (Glass and Strang 1991). This separation of the training function from the provision of client services can be argued to have increased the problems experienced by CDT members in adopting a consultancy role.

With the demise of the RDTUs there continues to be a separation of the training from the clinical function. Issues of role legitimacy have become increasingly emphasized by the more tightly defined roles of Community Mental Health Teams (CMHTs) which have increasingly restricted services on offer to people with severe and enduring mental health problems. People with substance misuse problems are referred on to specialist substance misuse services as a matter of course. Dually diagnosed patients may be offered 'shared care' but substance-related work (such as community detoxification) is still seen as exclusively the province of the specialist. Within Social Services a similar ethos exists in the majority of areas. Clients of the Probation Service are increasingly served by specific diversion from custody/arrest-referral schemes, which are often based within the non-statutory sector. There appears to be little recognition amongst service managers that social and health care workers should be working with their client's drug mis-use as well as the specific difficulties which led them to present to the particular agency (e.g. childcare/depression/offending).

In the absence of any legitimization of a more holistic approach and with substance misuse training low on the priority list it seems unlikely that the original consultancy role intended for CDTs will ever come to fruition. The need to enlist the resources of generic workers, however, remains self-evident. It is also clear that the manner in which this was originally attempted failed. This was due to a complex interaction of factors, some related to the lack of operational clarity, and support offered to the CDTs in carrying out such an ambitious agenda, but mainly related to the pressure of demand for specialist services at a time when mainstream mental health services were becoming more rigorous in their service specifications and the number of people with drug problems was growing.

Co-ordination of services

The ACMD in 1982 suggested that Community Drug Teams should play a pivotal role in the co-ordination of services for individual drug misusers. The reality of much CDT work is that the worker is more likely to be involved in some ephemeral activity which may be grandly titled 'liaison' but does not really constitute 'co-ordination'. Brown (1986) has argued that a team's ability or inability to co-ordinate services will be reflected in the number of service resources that the team itself controls. Teams with limited control over resources become involved in liaison rather than coordination because they are predominantly involved in mediation between client and services rather than actual direction of clients to available services. Most CDTs commanded few resources and their ability to co-ordinate care was often limited.

The continuing development of the Care Programme Approach (CPA) (Health of the Nation Key Area Handbook for Mental Illness, 1994; Effective Care Co-ordination in Mental Health, 1999, An Audit Pack for

Monitoring the Care Programme 2001b) has provided a framework with the potential for care co-ordination by the CDT. As a case management mechanism its introduction has resulted in significant improvements in co-ordination. The opportunities that the CPA structure continues to present are outlined in 'Models of Care' (2002). This document, which carries the status of a National Service Framework, outlines a new model of working, which again seeks to involve generic workers but in a much more targeted way, within a clearly structured framework.

Problems encountered by the original CDT model

The engagement of generic workers, particularly GPs, in the early identification and provision of services to drug users, the direct provision of services themselves, and the co-ordination and development of the overall pattern of service provision, were all seen as part of the original remit of the CDT. In practice the majority of teams quickly came to spend the majority of their time in face-to-face contact with clients leading to the re-creation of the specialist at the local level. Whilst there have been a small number of CDTs who obtained good co-operation from the broad mass of local GPs (Strang et al. 1992) the majority of CDTs have only been able to identify small numbers of local GPs willing to work with their clients. These GPs have then become seen as local 'specialists' whose case-loads have grown as colleagues have offloaded their drug-using patients. This re-creation of the specialist service, albeit in more accessible and 'user-friendly' form than previously, was a failure of the original plan.

The centrality of the consultancy role in the original CDT model related not only to a more appropriate location of services but also to the large scale of the problem to be tackled and the benefits of early identification. The recommendations were based, however, on a model of care in which generic workers were seen as being easily able and willing, with support, to meet the needs of the client for services. The often chaotic nature of the client group and the complexity of needs that were often presented made this seem increasingly less realistic for generic health and social care workers, particularly within a climate where their own services were becoming increasingly rigorous about their own service specifications.

Through the 1990s CDTs came under increasing pressure with the rise in methadone maintenance and became increasingly restricted to medical model interventions such as detoxification, prescribing and medication management. As drug counselling became increasingly provided from within the voluntary sector, specialist input itself became increasingly fragmented, with the local knowledge of the CDT becoming increasingly focused on the provision and demand for specific medical interventions. The role of CDTs became increasingly narrowly defined, within the context of a broader pattern of services.

The eventual emergence of a more comprehensive range and pattern of services

As the role of the CDT became narrower, there were however encouraging signs that many of the broader organizational and policy issues which had led to the problems in operationalizing the original model were beginning to be acknowledged and tackled by policy makers and planners. Problems with effectively engaging people in services (Modernising Mental Health Services 1998), developing effective partnership working between different agencies (Mental Health National Service Framework 1999) and the need for a structured system of care planning (Effective Care Co-ordination 1999) were all prominent themes of Guidance to mental health services issued in the 1990s. In retrospect, it seems naïve that the CDT had been expected to find unilateral solutions to systems problems that were only beginning to be recognized at the point when teams were being set up.

The introduction of Drug Action Teams in 1995 (Tackling Drugs Together, 1995) recognized that the role of service co-ordination and planning is a substantial one which needs to be located at the proper level. Drug Action Teams are multi-agency policy and implementation teams, responsible for implementing drug policy, planning, multi-agency training and service development. They commission services rather than trying to deliver them. Additionally, the establishment in 2001 of an explicit drugs National Treatment Agency (NTA) as a special health authority within the NHS is further evidence of the intention to give more firm central direction to the planned further expansion of drug services.

Other guidance and practice standards specific to drug services have also been forthcoming:

*   Report of an independent review of drug treatment services in England (Task Force to Review Services for Drug Misusers 1996)
*   Purchasing effective treatment and care for drug misusers: guidance for health authorities and social services departments (Department of Health 1997)
*   Drug misuse and dependence – guidelines for clinical management (Department of Health 1999)
*   Commissioning standards: drug and alcohol treatment and care (SMAS 1999)
*   QuADS: Organizational standards for alcohol and drug treatment services (DrugScope and Alcohol Concern 1999)

The documents are now finally establishing the various organizational frameworks and requirements which were missing. The previous lack of those frameworks undoubtedly contributed to major practical problems and made the failure of the original CDT model almost inevitable. Too much in short was expected from the CDT and its workers, and the response from most of the teams was a narrowing of role in accordance with what local needs could realistically be met with the resource available.

Possible future 'Models of Care'

One important aspect of the CDT's originally envisaged role which is still unresolved is how best to utilize the input of generic workers. A structure to enable this is provided in Models of Care (2002) that outlines different responsibilities for each agency involved with people with substance misuse problems. Models of Care explicitly recognizes some of the problems that require to be faced in the provision of a comprehensive network of services.

> to date, the substance misuse field has been characterised by substantial geographical variations in the availability, structure and processes of treatment and the outcomes achieved. There has been limited consensus about the essential components of specialist substance misuse services and limited recognition of the importance of links with other health, social care and criminal justice agencies. The Models of Care project aims to move towards consensus.
>
> (Department of Health 2002)

In proposing a consensus on care pathways signed up to by all parties it is seeking to establish a level of role legitimacy amongst generic workers which has so far remained elusive. What is being asked for, however, is far more clearly specified than has previously been the case and the implementation of policy guidance is being far more closely monitored.

Conclusion

More than 20 years have passed since the Maudsley Alcohol Pilot Project noted that providing generic workers with an account of the size of the problem and exhorting them to respond was not enough. These generic workers, often located in primary care, needed then, and still now need, to feel confident about their role legitimacy and role adequacy and to receive support in carrying out the required task if therapeutic commitment is to be obtained. It is necessary for the reasons for their previous failure to engage to be understood and to be worked through. The responsibility for this no longer lies with the CDT alone. Wider ownership of this challenge is required. There is now a clear need for another step forward.

References

ACMD (Advisory Council on the Misuse of Drugs) (1982). Report on treatment and rehabilitation. HMSO, London.

Advisory Committee on Alcoholism (1978). The pattern and range of services for problem drinkers. Department of Health and Social Security and Welsh Office, London.

Alien, G. (1983). Informal networks of care: issues raised by Barclay. *Journal of Social Work*, 13, 417–33.

Audit Commission for Local Authorities in England and Wales (1986). Making a reality of community care. HMSO, London.

Baldwin, S. (1987). Old wine in old bottles: why Community Alcohol Teams will not work. In *Helping the problem drinker: new initiatives in community care* (ed. T. Stockwell and S. Clement), pp. 158–71. Croom Helm, London.

Baldwin, S., Baser, C. and Pinker, A. A. (1986). The emperor's new community services. *Nursing Times – Community Outlook*, 12 February, pp. 6–8.

Barclay Report (1982). *Social workers: their role and tasks*. Bedford Square Press, London.

Brown, S. (1986). Community mental handicap teams: organisation, operation and outcomes. Report to DHSS. Department of Health, London.

Buning, E. (1990). The role of harm-reduction programmes in curbing the spread of HIV by drug injectors. In *AIDS and drug misuse: the challenge for policy and practice in the 1990s* (ed. J. Strang and G. V. Stimson), pp. 153–61. Routledge, London.

Campaign for Mental Handicap (1982). Teams for mentally handicapped people. Campaign for Mentally Handicapped People, London.

Cartwright, A. (1980). The attitudes of helping agents towards the alcoholic client: the influence of experience, support, training and self-esteem. *British Journal of Addiction*, 75, 413–31.

Clement, S. (1987). The Salford experiment: an account of the Community Alcohol Team approach. In *Helping the problem drinker: new initiatives in community care* (ed. T. Stockwell and S. Clement), pp. 121–44. Croom Helm, London.

Clement, S. (1989). The Community Drug Team: lessons from alcohol and handicap services. In *Treating drug abusers* (ed. G. Bennett), pp. 171–89. Routledge, London.

Cranfield, S. and Dixon, A. (1990). Drug training, HIV and AIDS in the 1990s: a guide for training professionals. Health Education Authority, London.

Department of Health (1997). Purchasing effective treatment and care for drug misusers: guidance for health authorities and social services departments. London. The Stationery Office.

Department of Health (1998). Modernising Mental Health Services: Safe, Sound and Supportive, London, HMSO.

Department of Health (1999). Mental Health National Service Frameworks: Modern Standards and Service Models, London, HMSO.

Department of Health (1999). Drug misuse and dependence – guidelines for clinical management. London. Department of Health.

Department of Health (1999). Effective Care Co-ordination in Mental Health. Modernising the Care Programme Approach. London. The Stationery Office.

Department of Health (2001a). The Mental Health Policy Implementation Guide, London, The Stationery Office.

Department of Health (2001b). An Audit Pack for Monitoring the Care Programme (http://doh.gov.uk/mentalhealth/auditpack.htm).

Department of Health (2002). Models of Care for substance misuse treatment. Report for Consultation (http://www.nta.nhs.uk/).

DrugScope and Alcohol Concern (1999). *QuADS: Organisational standards for alcohol and drug treatment services.* London. DrugScope/Alcohol Concern.

Glass, I. B. and Strang, J. (1991). Professional training in substance abuse: the UK experience. In *International handbook of addiction behaviour* (ed. I. B. Glass), pp. 333–40. Routledge, London.

Health of the Nation Key Area Handbook for Mental Illness (2nd Edition) (1994). HMSO, London.

House of Commons Social Services Committee (1985). Second Report from the Social Services Committee – Community Care with special reference to adult mentally ill and mentally handicapped people. HMSO, London.

Incichen, B. and Russell, J. A. O. (1980). Mental handicap and community care – the viewpoint of the general practitioner. Mental Handicap Studies Research Report No. 4. University of Bristol, Department of Mental Health.

MacGregor, S. (1994). Promoting new services: the Central Funding Initiative and other mechanisms. In *Heroin addiction and drug policy. The British System*, (ed. J. Strang and M. Gossop). Oxford University Press, Oxford.

MacGregor, S., Ettore, B., Coomber, R., Crosier, A. and Lodge, H. (1991). Drug services in England and the impact of the Central Funding Initiative, ISDD Research Monograph No. 1. Institute for the Study of Drug Dependence, London.

Maudsley Alcohol Pilot Project (1975). Designing a comprehensive community response to problems of alcohol abuse. Report to the Department of Health and Social Security, London.

National Development Group for the Mentally Handicapped (1980). Improving the quality of services for mentally handicapped people: a checklist of standards. Department of Health and Social Security, London.

Schneider, J., Davis, P., Nazum, W. and Bennett, G. (1989). The community drug team: current practice. In *Treating drug abusers* (ed. G. Bennett). Routledge, London.

Shaw, S., Cartwright, A., Spratley, T. and Harwin, J. (1978). *Responding to drinking problems.* Croom Helm, London.

Stockwell, T. and Clement, S. (1988). Community Alcohol Teams: a review of studies evaluating their effectiveness with special reference to the experience of other community teams. Report to Department of Health, London.

Strang, J. (1989). A model service: turning the generalist on to drugs. In *Drugs & British Society* (ed. S. MacGregor), pp. 143–69. Routledge, London.

Strang, J. (1991). Organization of services: drugs. In *International handbook of addiction behaviour* (ed. I. B. Glass), pp. 283–91. Routledge, London.

Strang, J. and Clement, S. (1994). The introduction of Community Drug Teams across the UK. In *Heroin addiction and drug policy. The British System* (ed. J. Strang and M. Gossop). Oxford University Press, Oxford.

Strang, J., Donmall, M., Webster, A., Abbey, J. and Tantam, D. (1991). A bridge not far enough: community drug teams and doctors in the North Western Region 1982–1986. ISDD Research Monograph No. 3. Institute for the Study of Drug Dependence (ISDD), London.

Strang, J., Smith, M. and Spurrell, S. (1992). The community drug team: data and analysis. *British Journal of Addiction*, 87, 169–78.

Substance Misuse Advisory Service (1999). Commissioning standards: drug and alcohol treatment and care. London, Health Advisory Service.

Tantam, D., Donmall, M., Webster, A. and Strang, J. (1993). Can general practitioners and general psychiatrists be expected to look after drug misusers? Results from evaluation of a non-specialist treatment policy in the northwest of England. *British Journal of General Practice*, 43, 470–4.

Task Force to Review Services for Drug Misusers (1996). Report of an independent review of drug treatment services in England. London, Department of Health.

UKADCU (1998). Tackling Drugs to Build a Better Britain. The government's 10 year strategy for tackling drugs misuse. London, The Stationery Office.

U.K. Home Office (1995). Tackling Drugs Together: a Strategy for England 1995–1998. London: Home Office.

Wistow, G. and Wray, K. (1986). CMHTs service delivery and service development: the Nottinghamshire way approach. In *Community Mental Handicapped Teams: theory and practice* (ed. G. Grant, S. Humphreys and M. Magrath). British Institute of Mental Handicap Conference Services.

Chapter 9

The coming of age of oral methadone maintenance treatment in the UK in the 1990s

Michael Farrell and Duncan Raistrick

Introduction

Practitioners visiting the UK from almost any other country in the world react to the UK approach to methadone treatment with a mixture of bemused critique, incredulity and a little envy. The curiosity is that the so-called British System, the origins of which are described in many chapters in this book, allows doctors an enormous amount of discretion in the way that they prescribe substitute drugs, usually methadone, and whether or not they associate their prescribing with some form of psycho-social therapy. Not surprisingly there is huge variation in the management of substitute prescribing and the UK style of working is often quite different to that reported in research papers from other countries. The Department of Health *Drug Misuse and Dependence – Guidelines on Clinical Management* (1999) goes a long way towards requiring a more regulated approach while at the same time preserving legitimate clinical freedoms. Just as most people in the general population have very definite opinions about drug use and drug users, so too do prescribers and the counsellors or therapists with whom they work. The visitor to the UK is likely to detect an absence of consensus on the purpose of methadone prescribing, or in other words treatment outcome goals, and it is unsurprising, therefore, that controversy and mis-information confuse the way that methadone programmes are defined and managed.

Methadone treatment is probably one of the most widely researched interventions in the addiction field and it follows that the benefits are well documented. In the UK the National Treatment Outcome Research Study (Gossop *et al.*, 1999), usually known as NTORS, has produced similar findings to many other studies from around the world. Typical findings are that in the substance misuse domain there are marked reductions in opiate use, reductions in the use of other illicit drugs notably including cocaine, and more variable but usually less dramatic reductions in alcohol and licit drug use; in the health domain there are dramatic reductions in high risk behaviours such as injecting, sharing needles and syringes, reduced rates of HIV and hepatitis, reduction in accidental overdosing, and improvements in mental state; in the social domain there are marked reductions in criminal activity, significant increases in employment and improved relationships. There is no doubt that there are benefits from methadone substitution; however, it is the detail that matters and the reader must exercise caution in comparing one type of methadone treatment with another. Methadone programmes are set up to achieve different objectives and even where the objectives are the same programmes have different characteristics and differ in overall quality of delivery. It is very easy to start prescribing methadone and see immediate improvements in the well-being of most patients, but what really matters is how the prescription is managed in the medium to long term.

The terminology of substitute prescribing is imprecise and sometimes misleading. The key issue is to understand that programmes are primarily driven by one of two major objectives – namely supporting *health or social policy*, on the one hand, and *treatment for the individual*, on the other hand. Unfortunately these two major objectives are often at odds with each other and can cause difficulty for the inexperienced prescriber. Methadone maintenance and low threshold methadone programmes are usually associated with the former objective and methadone reduction with the latter. A loose hierarchy exists between these different programmes:

(1)   As the name suggests, a *low threshold programme* is intended to have rapid and easy access with methadone prescribed more or less on demand. Such programmes are well known as a component of the Dutch and in particular Amsterdam drug policy (Buning and van Brussel, 1995) but the term does not have great currency in the UK. The low threshold programme is designed to deliver a harm reduction goal which has been defined in Amsterdam as being suitable for a drug user who is not capable or not willing to give up his or her drug use and who should be assisted in reducing the harm caused to themselves or others. In practice the parallel in the UK is with the many services who continue to work with users who are involved in ongoing polydrug use.

(2)   The *reducing methadone programme* is by far the most common approach used in primary care settings in the UK and also widely used within specialist services. These programmes are much more orientated towards individual treatment and typically have a medium-term goal of achieving abstinence. While the prescribers may see themselves as delivering individual treatment, such programmes are also expected to deliver health and social gains and can, as in the Glasgow experience (Gruer *et al.*, 1997), be driven by public health need.

(3)   *Methadone maintenance programmes*, like low threshold programmes, are aiming to achieve harm reduction objectives, but, unlike low threshold programmes, individuals typically graduate to maintenance after unsuccessful attempts at reduction and abstinence. In the UK, maintenance programmes

are predominantly supported by specialist services and include people on long-term injectable methadone and higher tariff substitute drugs.

What is important here is that different kinds of methadone programme deliver different outcomes for different kinds of people. So, the debate is not about 'Is heroin substitution better than methadone?' or 'Is maintenance better than reduction?' Rather it is about how best to integrate the variety of substitution packages that are known to be effective into a comprehensive local range of services.

Policy-driving practice

Over the past two decades there has been much debate about the funding of health services and the UK remains one of the countries in Europe with low per capita spending on health care. The use of primary care as a gatekeeper to secondary care services is regarded as conferring a level of efficiency of service utilisation that is unique. Despite the current limits to spending there continue to be debates about value for money, priorities in health care delivery and overall strategies for cost containment. These debates are similar to most industrialised nation debates on this subject. More recently, in recognition of the strong links between drug use and offending behaviour, there has been a substantial amount of new money invested in prisons, probation services and arrest referral schemes. This has not been matched by an equivalent investment in community and residential treatment programmes. The stated commitment of the Government, in the early 2000s, is to increase spending on the NHS and this is likely to benefit the spending on drug treatment to a significant extent.

Development of services

Prior to 1968 there were no clearly defined specialist services for drug misuse but after the Dangerous Drugs Act specialist services were established. There were three phases of service development. Ten per cent of current services were developed before 1970, 19 per cent mainly residential rehabilitation services in the 1970s, and the majority of services, 71 per cent, were established after the central funding initiative in 1984 (MacGregor, 1994). It has been argued that HIV and AIDS have stimulated the growth of the public health model of drug services (Stimson, 1995). Public health implications of HIV spread among drug users resulted in a range of proactive strategies with increased funding for the expansion of community drug services and the development of a wide network of needle exchange programmes. MacGregor and her colleagues, as part of a review for the Task Force (1996), reported that, in the decade since her previous review, there had been a widespread process of merger and consolidation of services (see also

Chapter 17, this volume, for discussion of the Task Force). By the mid-1990s there were over 475 services identified, 95 of which were residential or in-patient services and the rest were statutory or voluntary sector community-based drug agencies.

By the beginning of the new century, the key policy priorities had shifted once again. The major initiatives having moved from the public health sector to the criminal justice sector with crime reduction now driving the further investment in drug treatment services. While this may be the major current motor for service development, successful development necessitates that there be a good balance with equitable resource distribution between criminal justice and other treatment agencies based in the social and health sector of society.

Current situation of substitution treatment

Methadone prescribing services can be integrated into most settings, but typically belong to community-based multi-disciplinary teams who aim to provide psycho-social interventions ranging from brief interventions, motivational interviewing, cognitive behavioural and relapse prevention to addressing legal, housing and financial problems. Such activity may occur with community drug teams with their own medical staff or with shared care services linking into primary care. There has been a major emphasis on the development of shared care services and the promotion of primary care involvement in drug services over the last five years (Farrell and Gerada, 1997).

The UK has a network of methadone prescribing services with the majority being integrated into the mainstream of drug services and linked also to primary care services. Probably 95 per cent of methadone prescribed is done off-site by prescriptions being brought to community pharmacists, being dispensed by community pharmacists and being consumed at home. There is considerable geographic variation in the level of prescribing. Most of this activity occurs through community drug services which are in essence specialist services or secondary care services. There is a substantial amount of prescribing from general practitioners in association with these community drug teams. Up to 20 per cent of general practitioners may be involved in methadone prescribing but in some districts over 80 per cent of general practitioners still have no desire to be involved in substitute prescribing.

Guidelines and practice developments

There have been guidelines for the management of drug dependence since the mid-1980s. The original impetus of these guidelines, popularly referred to as the Orange Guidelines because of the colour of the original 1984 document and all subsequent documents, appears to have been prompted by the recommendations in the Treatment and Rehabilitation Report (ACMD,

1982) that there should be greater involvement of general practitioners and an associated concern expressed about the prescription of injectable drugs. These were advisory guidelines specifically aimed at general practitioners and recommended general practitioners to be involved in the short-term prescribing of substitute drugs as well as less complicated methadone maintenance. The next development occurred in the mid- to late 1980s when the rise in concern around HIV spread among injecting drug users caused a major review of drug treatment strategy and resulted in a significant shift to more harm reduction strategies. Thus the new Guidelines published in 1991 contained specific information and advice for injectors on how to clean injecting equipment in order to reduce the risk of transmission of HIV. The Health of the Nation (1990) public health strategy set targets for a reduction of sharing among injecting drug users and recommended that methadone maintenance treatment was an important tool for HIV prevention among injecting drug users. In the mid- to late 1980s the greatest concern about the spread of HIV among injecting drug users was in Edinburgh where high rates of HIV seroprevalence were reported (Robertson *et al.*, 1994; see also Chapter 10, Volume I, by Roy Robertson). This resulted in the establishment of the Edinburgh Community Problem Drug Advisory Service which rapidly established a network of methadone treatment clinics with a model for combining specialist input and primary care input (Greenwood, 1990, 1992).

In the early 1990s the Advisory Council on the Misuse of Drugs, in its Update Report on HIV and AIDS (1993), recommended an explicit emphasis on the benefits of methadone maintenance. Up until this point most official and advisory policy documents discussed methadone treatment but generally avoided the term methadone maintenance. In 1994 Farrell and co-authors published a major review of methadone maintenance treatment in the *British Medical Journal* which supported significant primary care involvement in methadone maintenance treatment (Farrell *et al.*, 1994). In Glasgow, the development of services was led by a public health model with a major emphasis on developing a network of supervised methadone consumption and other primary care inputs but limited specialist mental health input. In Northern Ireland, by contrast, professionals and policy makers continued to resist establishing methadone services and only a small number of individuals were treated with such medication. Throughout other parts of England and Wales many diverse models of shared care evolved (see Chapter 6, this volume, by Clare Gerada). In some settings where no specialist services existed, primary care developed models of shared care which involved minimal specialist support, and there were also other areas where specialist input was considerable and primary care involvement remained limited. In the absence of any clearly defined core service or clear consensus on the critical components of drug service delivery, the patterns of organisation, the patterns of service provision and the levels of skills of practitioners in the field all varied to such an extent that they were indicative of major quality control problems and major limitations in the overall standard of service provision in this field.

In the mid-1990s, a Task Force to Review the Effectiveness of Drug Services was established to review the then current treatment approaches. The Task Force was seen by the treatment field at the time (*Druglink*, 1994; and also see Chapter 17, this volume) as a vehicle which would dilute harm reduction approaches and in particular put a stop to drug substitution treatment. However, despite these reservations, the Task Force final report (1996) strongly supported the role for methadone maintenance treatment and supported further investment in treatment. This report was followed by guidelines for effective purchasing of drug treatment services which contained a strong endorsement for methadone maintenance treatment (Substance Misuse Advisory Service, 1999). The Task Force report recommended that the Clinical Guidelines for the management of Drug Dependence be updated. A working group published a completely reworked version of the Orange Guidelines in 1999 and recommended a move towards tighter monitoring and supervision of methadone – particularly in the early phases of treatment. A key issue was that recommended practice would minimise the diversion of prescribed psychoactive drugs and would reduce both fatal and non-fatal opioid overdoses. These guidelines placed considerable emphasis on the role of shared care and primary care services. Detailed approaches to dose induction and safety aspects of methadone prescribing were emphasised and three levels of skill were defined – the 'generalist', the 'specialist generalist' and the 'specialist' – and a training approach to these skill levels was outlined. Subsequently it has been recommended that new legislation be enacted to restrict the prescribing of injectable medication and some other medication to prescribers who are specialists and are authorised licence holders and this process is currently undergoing a broad consultation process.

In the late 1990s, with the advantage of being driven by the National Drug Strategy, methadone treatment was beginning to attract a more sophisticated assessment of its use and purpose; targeting of suitably adapted programmes began to climb the commissioning agenda. For example, shared care between specialists and primary care was becoming accepted as the norm, and treatment services collaborated with probation services through Drug Treatment and Testing Orders. Following a period of pilot projects the DTTOs were rolled out across the treatment system in England (for further discussion, see Chapter 16, this volume, by Emily Finch and Mike Ashton).

Primary Care involvement

Shared care participation has been identified as an important development area (Task Force, 1996; Clinical Guidelines, 1999). Though limited in number, well-implemented initiatives show that it is possible to deliver opioid maintenance treatment in a general practice setting for many patients, provided there is an ongoing case management and active collaboration with a specialist service. The importance of delivering services to drug users in non-metropolitan areas, where specialist services may have limited capacity, underscores the importance of further developing reduction and maintenance treatments. There is a major policy emphasis on expanding primary care involvement in the management of drug dependence. This includes strategies to provide further financial support for general practitioner involvement and provision of financial support to develop shared care strategies between primary care and specialist services.

The task of the late 1990s and early part of the new century was to create significantly greater treatment capacity. It was viewed that this could only be achieved through greater involvement of primary care. A national training programme followed on from the Clinical Guidelines to support further development of General Practitioners with appropriate training in the management of drug dependence in Primary Care. There continues to be a push to expand the involvement of general practitioners.

Prisons

There has been a considerable expansion in the growth of detoxification for prisoners but only a limited amount of methadone maintenance in prisons. Overall, surveys indicate that half of the women and a third of the men who were identified as drug dependent in the year before prison received help for their drug problem during that time. Also a substantial proportion of those in the sentenced population had some contact with helping agencies during their prison stay. Those with opiate dependence were more likely to receive help in the community and also more likely to get help in prison but dependent stimulant users also reported significant levels of access to help within prison settings.

Substitute prescribing is one of the commonest forms of treatment delivered by community treatment agencies and yet there is still only a low level of continuity between community methadone treatment and prison methadone treatment. Data indicate that, for those who are sentenced, there are reasonable levels of contact with outside specialist agencies. Service expansion for drug users within prisons has changed significantly in the recent past with the development of a range of pilot treatment programmes and the publication of the Prison Service's Corporate Plan (Prison Service Drug Strategy, 1995). There is a strong recognition of the links between acquisitive criminality and drug dependence and recent work on a national treatment cohort (Gossop et al., 1998) identified high rates of active offending among those newly entering drug treatment services. There has been recognition for some time that there is a considerable drug problem associated with the prison setting. The prisons continue to face a major challenge in putting in place appropriate responses. Since 1996 Mandatory Drug Testing in prisons has reported that roughly 4 per cent of prisoners test positive for opiates across the prison estate. Strategies to tackle this effectively have yet to be put in place.

Patterns of prescribing and dispensing among practitioners

Given the nature of the clinical activity and the limited amount of central data gathering on this activity much of the actual practice of doctors can only be inferred from indirect research data. This section describes the results of surveys and individual research projects rather than any form of central audit information. The Department of Health Clinical Guidelines (1999) were particularly concerned to reduce the possibility of diversion of prescribed medicines as well as looking for ways to increase compliance with treatment and thereby enhance the beneficial impact of treatment.

There is a small private treatment sector, almost entirely restricted to London, which mainly focuses on the prescribing of injectable methadone and amphetamines because of the limited prescribing of these drugs within mainstream services. While these private services constitute a very small part of the overall provision they have a significant impact on London-based services. This was explored by Strang and Sheridan (2001).

Because of the permissive way that the UK allows prescribing and dispensing of substitution medication, there is a major amount of diversion of prescribed medication and a large black market for methadone where the commonly prescribed oral syrup form of methadone costs 10 pounds sterling per 100 mg, and ampoules of methadone and heroin are correspondingly more expensive (see Fountain et al., 2000; Fountain and Strang, 2003). To date, drug diversion has not been a major political issue but there are rising numbers of first treatment episodes for methadone only and there have been anecdotal reports of deaths from recreational methadone use. However, a continued rise in the number of opiate- and methadone-related deaths has resulted in a degree of alarm around this issue and calls for more supervision of prescribed methadone. Fountain et al. (2000) described a framework for consideration of diversion of pharmaceutical products and based on anthropological field work indicated that any consideration of the organisation and delivery of drug treatment services that involve prescribing psychoactive medication needs to take account of the dynamic of prescribed drug diversion in how the services are planned.

Pharmacy activity

In the UK there have been two comparable surveys of pharmacy activity throughout England and Wales, the first in 1988 (Glanz et al., 1989) and the second in 1995 (Sheridan *et al.*, 1997). Sheridan *et al.* (1997) found a large increase in the percentage of community pharmacies involved in the provision of services for drug misusers – 23 per cent in 1988 rising to 50 per cent in 1995. Of 3,693 methadone prescriptions being dispensed from the selected pharmacies in the 1995 study details of the type and dose of methadone prescribed and the dispensing arrangements were collated. Across the whole sample 79 per cent of all prescriptions were for oral liquid methadone, 11 per cent were for tablets and 9 per cent were for methadone ampoules (Strang *et al.*, 1996).

Guidelines from the UK Departments of Health advise doctors to instruct the dispensing pharmacist to provide methadone in instalments – for example, daily dispensing. The national Pharmacy Survey (described in the preceding paragraph) found that more than one-third (37 per cent) of all prescriptions examined in the study were for weekly or fortnightly pick-up, with 38 per cent being for daily pick-up. Furthermore, general practitioners prescribed with longer intervals between pick-ups than hospital doctors. Tablets and ampoules were less likely to be dispensed on a daily basis. Across the UK there was considerable variation in dispensing arrangements so, for example, the proportion of prescriptions dispensed daily was 16 per cent in one region compared to 65 per cent in another.

Doses of methadone dispensed varied according to the type of methadone prescribed with oral mixtures being most likely to be prescribed at the lower dose range. This would appear to indicate that despite evidence for greater benefit from higher dose oral methadone maintenance that practice in the mid- to late 1990s continued to err to the lower dose range and probably also indicates that a substantial amount of clinical activity continues to be 'maintenance to detoxification'. However, in the absence of more specific data, these comments are speculative in nature. Where the daily dose of methadone was less than 50 mg, 71.2 per cent of prescriptions were for oral methadone; where the daily dose of methadone was 100 mg or more only 1.5 per cent of prescriptions were for oral methadone. Private prescriptions were significantly more likely than NHS ones to be for tablets or ampoules, to be for substantially higher doses and to be collected on a weekly or fortnightly basis. Eighty per cent of all private prescriptions were from the London area.

There is considerable variation in the balance between injectable and oral methadone prescribing with some regions reporting up to 10 per cent of prescribing in injectable form and some regions reporting minimal injectable prescribing. There is no regulation or limitation on practitioners in determining the balance between oral and injectable prescribing. Heroin prescribing is done within the specialist services where, alongside other influences, the cost has effectively limited the amount of such prescribing. There is consideration and exploration of further studies to evaluate injectable prescribing. Two studies have recently been completed. The first a descriptive outcome study of people on injectable methadone and diamorphine reported positive outcomes (Metrebian *et al.*, 1998) and the second is a small pilot randomised study of injectable versus oral methadone (Strang *et al.*, 2000) which found, with a small cohort randomised to either oral and injectable treatment, the six-month outcomes were not markedly different.

Alternatives to methadone

Methadone is generally taken as the gold standard reference for substitute prescribing because its properties include: (i) a long half-life ensuring suppression of withdrawal and craving throughout a 24-hour period from single daily dosing; (ii) a modest potency of effect as compared to other opiates favoured by drug users; (iii) slow absorption rate when taken orally; (iv) effective blockade of opiate receptors at methadone plasma levels in excess of 0.6 nmol/L. This cluster of characteristics is inherently stabilising and well suited to long-term prescribing; however, it is not uncommon for users to complain of feeling 'flat' when taking methadone. It is also the case that the very properties that make methadone suitable for stabilisation make it a more difficult drug to withdraw from than shorter-acting opiates. In addition to the problems experienced by users there are also concerns about the safety profile of methadone.

Methadone deaths in the early stage of treatment are being reported with increasing frequency. Australian research indicates that risk of death in the first weeks of methadone treatment is substantial and requires skilled and careful management to minimise this risk (Capelhorn, 1998). Some services have established dose induction services and the role of such services require further exploration.

There are alternatives to methadone. Buprenorphine has been extensively studied as an alternative substitution therapy to methadone (Ling *et al.*, 1998). Buprenorphine has the benefit of an improved safety profile compared to methadone, an easier withdrawal and high user acceptability. There have been concerns about using buprenorphine in the UK because of earlier epidemics of intravenous abuse of the painkiller Temgesic (buprenorphine that was marketed for the purpose of analgesic medication). In fact the misuse of Temgesic was generally at dose levels that are at the lower end of what is now considered appropriate for addiction substitution treatment and so the history should not necessarily obstruct the introduction of buprenorphine to the UK. There are currently a number of studies looking at how buprenorphine fits into the UK context both for the purposes of substitution and detoxification. By 2001 high-dose formulations of buprenorphine were approved for addiction treatment and thereby it became available as an alternative choice for either detoxification or maintenance treatment of opioid dependence. LAAM, a long-acting opioid agonist with a two to three day profile of activity, was briefly available but was withdrawn because of concerns about cardiac toxicity.

Psycho-social components of treatment

Most studies of methadone programmes point to the need for an accompanying psycho-social therapy. In the UK the level of variation in psycho-social input appears to be profound and cannot be justified by differing client needs. It is likely that in the future commissioners of services will require providers of methadone programmes to define the nature of the accompanying psycho-social therapies. In some situations the prescriber will also be competent to deliver a psycho-social therapy but often the two tasks will be divided. In the latter case it is essential that the doctor and therapist have an agreed model of understanding addictive behaviour in order that communication is possible and shared goals can be progressed. The most efficient and effective way of delivering treatment is within the one agency, usually doctors and other therapists belonging to a specialist NHS unit or an addiction therapist working as part of a primary care team; shared care models of working are also important and will be increasingly common but they are organisationally more difficult and always at risk of becoming overly bureaucratic.

It is often the case that work with opiate users involves multi-agency collaboration which may well include the criminal justice system, psychiatric services, HIV and hepatitis specialists, housing and other social care agencies. As clients move between these agencies it is important to avoid duplicating effort and giving conflicting treatment messages. It is highly desirable to have local protocols describing the roles of and flow between different agencies in order that the limited resources available are used in an effective way. What should usually be avoided is the situation where a client is attending two addiction agencies simultaneously; it is likely that at best there will be some duplication of effort and at worst there will be no cohesion to the treatment plan.

Substitute prescribing should always be enhanced by a psycho-social input which might be quite minimal and delivered by the prescriber, say in the case of methadone maintenance, or might be quite intensive and delivered by an addiction therapist, say in the case of a reducing programme aiming to achieve abstinence within a timescale around six months. The cost of psycho-social services can be considerable and so it follows that programmes should seek to deliver the optimal package. There are no UK studies that have looked at this specific point but in the United States McLellan et al. (1993) have investigated this very issue. McLellan and colleagues found that methadone alone, even at a minimum dose of 60 mg, was only effective for a minority of clients; methadone enhanced by a structured, cognitive behavioural therapy delivered significantly better outcomes and this, which they described as a standard treatment, was improved upon further by the inclusion of a whole gamut of counselling and support services. Further analysis of the cost effectiveness found that, at 12 months, the annual cost per abstinent client was $16,485, $9,804 and $11,818 for the low, intermediate and high levels of intervention respectively. Other studies have also found that adding more intensive therapy brings about more change but this has to be set against an equally consistent finding that most change in therapy occurs within the first three months and the more intensive therapy delivers diminishing outcome returns. While the treatment benefits may facilitate continuing natural change processes and be good value for money, there are clearly limits to both intensity and duration of therapy.

The National Treatment Outcome Research Study (NTORS) was a pragmatic trial that followed the outcomes of patients attending for different kinds of treatment programmes, namely: in-patient; residential; methadone maintenance; and methadone reduction. In this kind of trial little can be said about the effectiveness of the different kinds of treatment since each programme is likely to attract patients with different characteristics; however, this kind of research does show up what happens to patients attending real world services as opposed to services that are distorted by the requirements of a random controlled trial. NTORS (Department of Health, 1998) concluded that treatment should be seen as a process in which the patient takes an active role rather than a discreet event delivered by professionals. In NTORS, 75 per cent of treatments involved substitute prescribing, 19 per cent of participants had attended Narcotics Anonymous, more than half had been to a street agency, and they were regular users of health and social care resources. NTORS estimated that the total cost of drug use by the study clients was 14.3 million pounds and 81 per cent of this was made up from victim costs and criminal justice system costs. At one year follow-up the amount spent by addicts on purchasing drugs was reduced by approximately 75 per cent or an overall reduction of costs was 12,650 pounds sterling per annum per person. From these data NTORS calculated that for every one pound spent on drug misuse treatment there were savings of three pounds from reduced victim costs and reduced demand on the criminal justice system. In addition to this there are savings to the health service and social care services. Overall, it seems fair to say that treatment is good value for money but what is more difficult is to define what kind of treatment, and in particular what substitution regimens, give the best value.

In the UK, clinical governance has become all important in the management of provider agencies. Services face a serious dilemma in that it is very difficult to recruit staff who have received accredited training in addiction work but services also recognise that the business of delivering an effective treatment requires skilled therapists. Luborsky et al. (1985) compared the effectiveness of two manual guided therapies, supportive expressive and cognitive behavioural, combined with para-professional drug counselling. Both structured therapies did better than drug counselling alone but most striking were the differences between the effectiveness of different therapists. For example, the best therapist achieved a positive change in drug use of 34 per cent compared to a worsening of drug use by 14 per cent for the least good therapist; on the measure of psychiatric state the differences were 82 per cent improvement against 1 per cent deterioration. Differences of this magnitude are sufficient to obscure differences in main treatment effects. This and other studies suggest that not only must therapists be adequately trained but their performance is likely to be improved by using manual-based therapies and by checking on adherence to these therapies – for example by video recording of therapy sessions.

It is probably in the field of vocational rehabilitation for clients and general training for their subsequent job-seeking that the methadone treatment field in the UK has singularly failed to date. For much of the 1980s, the poor jobs market made the prospect of having a real impact on returning to work a seriously challenging task. However, in the early twenty-first century, the jobs situation has changed considerably and there is a strong commitment from central government to encourage people back into the workplace. A number of projects on Dependence to Work have been developed but there are, as yet, no data available for their particular impact on individuals who have been long-term opiate-dependent. Such occupational rehabilitation activities have a potentially critical role to play in overall social rehabilitation and it is hoped that the literature on this subject will grow over the coming decade.

Conclusion

In the new century, opiate substitution treatment in the UK is beginning to diversify, with a significant growth in the use of buprenorphine as an alternative. Also the use of lofexidine in detoxification has provided a wider range of options for the management of opiate detoxification. Overall, substantial progress has been made. However, substantial problems still exist, with reports of long waiting lists for methadone treatment, and with many services operating at full capacity and unable to develop to meet the broader demands. The need for these services to link in with Criminal Justice agencies to provide treatment in the Criminal Justice System remains a major challenge.

Poor methadone treatment is still widespread in the UK. Four particularly disappointing aspects of today's British System will form the basis of the conclusion of this chapter. First, there is the continuing uncertainty over the issue of methadone dose, and whether high-dose maintenance should be actively encouraged: at present, it is still largely determined by the whim and inclination of the senior doctor and multi-disciplinary team of the individual agency. Second, there is the widespread ignorance of, and disregard for, the international evidence on the substantial influence of the psycho-social component of comprehensive care (for a review see Raistrick, 2003), and a reliance on what Strang and Tober (2003) described as just 'wishing well but doing badly': methadone maintenance programmes in the UK need to look at the gap between their impact and the greater impact in other countries and ask themselves why there is such a difference (Royal College of Psychiatrists and Physicians, 2000). Third, there are prisons, with their woefully inadequate level of actual provision of maintenance and other proper detoxification treatments, despite at least a decade of official guidance of at least adequate standards. And fourth, there is the continued low level of supervised methadone in both pharmacy and specialist service setting, and the contribution this makes to the uniquely British extent to which methadone is itself implicated in the figures on opiate overdose deaths. In the context of efforts to foster quality improvement and increase treatment compliance, it is essential to address these areas, so as to be able to support a competent partnership between primary care and secondary care services for the future provision of high-quality methadone maintenance treatment in tomorrow's 'British System'.

References

ACMD (1982). Treatment and Rehabilitation Report. Department of Health. HMSO, London.

ACMD (1993). AIDS and Drug Misuse: An Update. Department of Health. The Stationery Office, London.

Buning, E. and van Brussel, G. (1995). The effects of harm reduction in Amsterdam. *European Addiction Research*, 1, 92–8.

Capelhorn, J. (1998). Deaths in the first two weeks of maintenance treatment in New South Wales in 1994: identifying cases of iatrogenic methadone toxicity. *Drug and Alcohol Review*, 17, 9–18.

Department of Health (1999). *Drug Misuse and Dependence – Guidelines on Clinical Management*, The Stationery Office, London.

Farrell, M. and Gerada, C. (1997). Drug misusers: whose business is it? *British Medical Journal*, 315, 559–60.

Farrell, M., Ward, J., Mattick, R., Hall, W., Stimson, G. V., des Jarlais, D., Gossop, M. and Strang, J. (1994). Methadone maintenance treatment in opiate dependence: a review. *British Medical Journal*, 309, 997–1001.

Fountain, J. and Strang, J. (2003). The illicit market in methadone: the play, the plot and the players. In G. Tober and J. Strang (eds) *Methadone Matters*. Dunitz, London.

Fountain, J., Griffiths, P., Farrell, M., Gossop, M. and Strang, J. (2000). Diversion of prescribed drugs by drug users in treatment: analysis of the UK market and new data from London. *Addiction*, 95, 393–406.

Gerada, C. and Farrell, M. (1998). Shared care. In R. Robertson (ed.) *Treating Drug Misuse in the Community*. Routledge, London.

Glanz, A., Byrne, C. and Jackson, P. (1989). Role of community pharmacies in prevention of AIDS among injecting drug misusers: findings of a survey in England and Wales. *British Medical Journal*, 299, 1076–9.

Gossop, M., Marsden, J. and Stewart, D. (1998). *NTORS at One Year: Changes in Substance Use, Health and Criminal Behaviour One Year after Intake*. Department of Health, London.

Gossop, M., Marsden, J., Stewart, D. and Rolfe, A. (1999). Treatment retention and one-year outcomes for residential programmes in England. *Drug Alcohol Dependence*, 57(2), 89–98.

Greenwood, J. (1990). Creating a new drug service in Edinburgh. *British Medical Journal*, 300, 587–9.

Greenwood, J. (1992). Persuading general practitioners to prescribe – good husbandry or a recipe for chaos? *British Journal of Addiction*, 87: 567–75.

Gruer, L., Wilson, P., Scott, R., Elliott, L., Macleod, J., Harden, K., Forrester, E., Hinshelwood, S., McNulty, H. and Silk, P. (1997). General practitioner centred scheme for treatment of opiate dependent drug injectors in Glasgow, *British Medical Journal*, 314, 1730–5.

Department of Health (1990). Health of the Nation. HMSO, London.

Ling, W., Charavastra, C., Collins, J. F. *et al.* (1998). Buprenorphine maintenance treatment of opiate dependence: a multicenter, randomised clinical trial, *Addiction*, 93, 475–86.

Luborsky, L., McLellan, A. T., Woody, G. E., O'Brien, C. P. and Auerbach, A. (1985). Therapist success and its determinants. *Archives of General Psychiatry*, 42, 602–11.

MacGregor, S. (1994). Promoting new services: the Central Funding Initiative and other mechanisms. In J. Strang and M. Gossop (eds) *Heroin Addiction and Drug Policy: The British System*. Oxford: Oxford University Press.

McLellan, A. T., Arndt, I. O., Metzger, D. S., Woody, G. E. and O'Brien, C. P. (1993). The effects of psychosocial services in substance abuse treatment, *Journal of the American Medical Association*, 269, 1953–9.

Metrebian, N., Shanahan, W., Well, S. B. and Stimson, G. (1998). Feasibility of prescribing injectable heroin and methadone to opiate-dependent drug users: associated health gains and harm reductions. *Medical Journal of Australia*, 168, 596–600.

News report (1994). Task force effectiveness of drug services, *Druglink*, September issue.

Prison Service Drug Strategy (1998). Tackling Drugs in Prison. London, HM Prison Service.

Raistrick, D. (2003). Psychosocial elements of methadone treatment. In G. Tober and J. Strang (eds) *Methadone Matters*. Dunitz, London.

Robertson, J. R., Ronald, P. J., Raab, J. M., Ross, G. M. and Parpia, T. (1994). Deaths, HIV infection, abstinence, and other outcomes in a cohort of injecting drug users followed up for 10 years. *British Medical Journal*, 309, 369–72.

Royal College of Psychiatrists and Physicians (2000). *Drugs: Dilemmas and Choices*. Gaskell, London.

Sheridan, J., Strang, J., Barber, N. and Glanz, A. (1996). Role of community pharmacies in relation to HIV prevention and drug misuse: finding from the 1995 national survey in England and Wales. *British Medical Journal*, 313: 272–4.

Sheridan, J., Strang, J., Taylor, C. and Barber, N. (1997). HIV prevention and drug treatment services for drug misusers: a national study of community pharmacists' attitudes and their involvement in service specific training. *Addiction*, 92, 1737–48.

Stimson, G. (1995). AIDS and injecting drug use in the United Kingdom, 1987–1993. The policy response and the prevention of an epidemic. *Social Science and Medicine*, 41, 699–716.

Strang, J. and Sheridan, J. (1998). National and regional characteristics of methadone prescribing in England and Wales: local analyses of data from the 1995 national survey of community pharmacies. *Journal of Substance Misuse*, 3, 240–6.

Strang, J. and Sheridan, J. (2001). Methadone prescribing to opiate addicts by private doctors: comparison with NHS practice in south-east England. *Addiction*, 96, 567–76.

Strang, J. and Tober, G. (2003). Methadone: universal panacea or pernicious poison? In G. Tober and J. Strang (eds) *Methadone Matters*. Dunitz, London.

Strang, J., Marsden, J., Cummins, M., Farrell, M., Finch, E., Gossop, M., Stewart, D. and Welch, S. (2000). Randomised trial of supervised injectable versus oral methadone maintenance: report on feasibility and six-month outcome. *Addiction*, 95: 1613–45.

Strang, J., Ruben, S., Farrell, M. and Gossop, M. (1994). Prescribing heroin and other injectable drugs. In J. Strang and M. Gossop (eds) *Heroin Addiction and Drug Policy: The British System*. Oxford: Oxford University Press.

Strang, J., Sheridan, J. and Barber, N. (1996). Prescribing injectable and oral methadone to opiate addicts: results from the 1995 national postal survey of community pharmacies in England and Wales. *British Medical Journal*, 313, 270–2.

Substance Misuse Advisory Service (1999). *Commissioning Standards Drugs and Alcohol Treatment and Care*, Health Advisory Service, London.

Task Force to Review Services for Drug Misusers (1996). Report of an Independent Review of Drug Treatment Services in England. London: Department of Health.

Chapter 10

Last call for injectable opiate maintenance

In pursuit of an evidence base for good clinical practice

Deborah Zador

(This chapter originally appeared in journal form as: Zador, D. (2001) Injectable opiate maintenance: is it good clinical practice? *Addiction*, 96: 547–553.)

This chapter reviews the current practice of injectable opiate treatment (IOT) in the UK, i.e. the 'British system' of prescribing injectable heroin and methadone, and considers some of the clinical and ethical issues it raises. There is only very limited research evidence supporting either the safety or effectiveness of IOT as practised in Britain. In particular there is almost no evaluation of long-term outcomes of IOT which is of potential concern given the possibility of some patients remaining indefinitely in IOT, the risk of vascular complications, and its higher cost compared with oral mainten-ance. It would be easy to assess this controversial intervention as in need of further research. However, striving towards best practice in IOT involves more than generating evidence. The likelihood of a patient receiving IOT in the UK appears to be influenced more by the personal inclinations of pre-scribers than by outcome data (if any), or identified community needs for access to IOT. Is this good clinical practice and is it sustainable? The British system needs to modernise itself, consistent with international paradigms of continuous quality improvement and with the NHS's own agenda of clinical governance.

The UK differs from most other countries by including injectable heroin and injectable methadone in its range of opiate substitution therapies for heroin-dependent users. A small number of licensed medical practitioners, usually specialists in drug dependence, can prescribe heroin to any depend-ent heroin user who is assessed to be suitable for this intervention. No licence is required for parenteral methadone. Currently, to the surprise of many addictions specialists and their patients, pharmaceutical heroin does not actually have an approval licence for treatment of opioid drug dependence, and parenteral methadone is not licensed for intravenous administration.

Britain has had a clinical experience with injectable opiate treatment (IOT) that is unsurpassed by other countries and of great interest to international drug services (for further historical account of injectable prescribing in the UK, see Chapter 1, this volume). Since at least the beginning of the twentieth century, doctors in Britain have been prescribing opioid drugs to their dependent patients. Following the release of the Rolleston report in 1926, medical practitioners were allowed to prescribe injectable opiates to addicts for the purpose of maintenance. In the 1920s and 1930s this was primarily morphine; however, during the 1960s this was supplanted by heroin as the profile of 'addict' changed from that of patients dependent on prescribed opiates to younger, illicit intravenous drug users. A substantial re-orientation of drug treatment occurred when provision of IOT shifted from individual doctors to specialist drug dependence units in 1968.

By the late 1970s, oral methadone became the predominant form of opioid maintenance treatment in response to the plethora of data emerging from the United States demonstrating the effectiveness of oral methadone maintenance treatment (MMT) and the results of local research undertaken by Hartnoll *et al.* (1980), which found inconclusive differences in outcome between oral methadone and injectable heroin. Currently, the option of IOT is infrequently exercised – less than 1.7 per cent of all prescriptions for treatment of opiate dependence are for heroin while injectable methadone accounts for about another 9 per cent (Strang *et al.* 1996). In the late 1990s, IOT became an even smaller part of the prescribing element of treating opiate addicts, with heroin prescribing remaining numerically static at about 500 patients (Metrebian *et al.* 2002), and with injectable methadone prescribing also remaining fairly static numerically, representing a reduction as a proportion of all methadone prescribing from the 9 per cent figure of the mid-1990s to only 4 per cent by 2001 (Strang and Sheridan 2003; and see Chapter 1, this volume).

The *Guidelines on Clinical Management* (UK Department of Health 1999) recommended that injectable opiates should only be prescribed to patients with long, complicated and intractable histories of opioid dependence, and/or who have 'failed' other forms of treatment including oral MMT, i.e. IOT should be an option of last resort. These *Guidelines* are vague and broad as they must be in the absence of comprehensive research and clinical evidence. For example, they include no recommendations on starting or maintenance doses of heroin. Therefore, their interpretation is at the discretion of the individual prescriber whose assessment and ongoing management of the patient is predominantly guided by prior experience with IOT.

However, the new 1999 *Guidelines* represent a policy response to the minimally regulated practice of IOT by acknowledging its occurrence and attempting to introduce guidelines to govern its practice. They recommend, as for oral MMT, the supervised administration of injectable heroin and methadone during initiation and stabilisation of treatment, if not longer. Presently in the UK injectable heroin is dispensed by community pharmacists and taken unsupervised as take-home doses.

There is a good deal of variation in the clinical practice of IOT. One study found the median maximum dose of heroin was 200 mg/day (Sell *et al.* 1997), while other studies reported mean doses ranging from 185 mg a day (SD = 15.7, range 150–200 mg) (Metrebian *et al.* 1998) to 295 mg/day (SD = 121 mg) (McCusker and Davies 1996). All these doses are substantially lower than those administered to subjects (mean dose: 509 mg/day, quartiles: 400, 480, 630 mg/day) in the Swiss heroin trials (Perneger *et al.* 1998). Interpretation of the British data is complicated by the virtually unevaluated practice of supplementing heroin prescriptions with injectable or oral methadone doses. There are also few data on the prescribing patterns of injectable methadone treatment (Strang *et al.* 1996; Strang and Sheridan 1998) and almost none on its effectiveness (Strang *et al.* 2000).

This chapter will contemplate some of the conundrums that the prescription of injectable opiates raises. It will begin by summarising the arguments for and against IOT then proceed with an examination of the legitimacy of these positions. Finally, as it is difficult to separate out a discussion of IOT in the UK from that of the British system, it will conclude with a discussion of the future of both. It will not review IOT as practised in other countries. For purposes of this chapter, IOT refers only to heroin and methadone while 'treatment' is broadly defined as a process of achieving a positive change in drug-using behaviour.

Arguments for injectable opiate prescribing in the UK

Advocates justify IOT on the grounds that it has a public health benefit and that it reduces harm. They contend that it decreases acquisitive crime and street heroin overdose, and that pharmaceutical heroin is of known purity and free of the contaminants or adulterants that are widely believed to be present in street heroin. Proponents of injectable heroin and methadone treatment argue that intervention reduces the spread of HIV, hepatitis B and C and other blood-borne viral diseases (BBVD). Injectable opiate treatment is believed to better attract and retain in treatment intractable heroin users who have rejected oral MMT or other interventions. Implicit in the last argument is the acceptance by IOT advocates of 'needle-fixation' as a legitimate indication for initiation of IOT. Finally, it is argued that if IOT is withheld from some heroin users they will either inject illicit opiates anyway or move onto more dangerous drugs and/or riskier behaviours.

Arguments against injectable opiate prescribing in the UK

Opponents of IOT respond that this treatment perpetuates injecting behaviour and that in the case of prescribed heroin it may postpone by years eventual abstinence from heroin. There is concern that prescribing injectable opiates might be associated with an increased incidence of deep venous thrombosis (DVT) as a consequence of injecting into (typically) the femoral veins ('the groins') following loss of venous access in the arms. Concern is also expressed about infection of venous and surrounding tissue. Opponents of IOT believe the maintenance of long-term intravenous injecting is contrary to the role of doctors to improve or maintain the physical health of their patients.

Objectors contend that IOT imparts to recipients of this treatment an impression that their 'needle-fixation' is indeed unmanageable and that they have been consigned to the 'scrap-heap' of untreatable patients. Alternatively IOT patients may confuse prescription of their parenteral opiates as a sanctioning or endorsement of their injecting behaviour by the prescriber. Finally, the option of IOT may provide some patients with a vested interest in a poor outcome while in oral MMT.

The evidence for and against injectable opiate prescribing in the UK

The few studies that have evaluated heroin maintenance treatment in the UK (Hartnoll *et al.* 1980; Battersby *et al.* 1992; Metrebian *et al.* 1998) reported reduced levels of crime among heroin-maintained patients as measured by self-report. However, even this reduction of criminal activity is unlikely to impact on the wider community because such a small proportion of the heroin-using population is prescribed heroin.

For heroin maintenance treatment to exert an impact at the population level on the negative social consequences of dependent heroin use such as crime would require, among other conditions, a substantial scaling-up in provision of this treatment (Hall 1999). Furthermore, the effectiveness of heroin maintenance demonstrated under the conditions of clinical trials may not be replicated if the same degree of quality is not maintained in its scaling-up (Hall 1999).

Finally, the diversion and sale of prescribed opiates on the black market is itself, of course, a criminal activity. Although the public apparently tolerates the current level of prescribed injectable opiates in the UK, it may not continue to do so if, in the event of a substantial expansion of this intervention, leakage onto the black market or other problems also increase.

The presumption that prescribed heroin of known purity reduces the risk of overdose is appealing but ignores the wealth of recent literature identifying the only moderate association between heroin purity and fatal heroin 'overdose' (Darke *et al.* 1999), the finding of the high frequency of polydrug use among cases of heroin-related deaths (Darke and Zador 1996; Risser *et al.* 2000), and other risk factors for overdose (Powis *et al.* 1999).

Injecting of prescribed opiates *per se* does not reduce the risk of BBVD infection among injecting drug users – rather, it is the use of clean needles, syringes and other equipment to inject street heroin, prescribed medications or any other drug. It may be argued, however, that IOT increases the opportunities for reinforcement of these harm reduction strategies.

The recent epidemic of deaths in Britain related to the injection of infected batches of heroin could be advanced as an argument for the prescription of pharmaceutical heroin but lethal pathogens are an uncommon contaminant of street heroin. Recent analyses of confiscated samples of heroin sold by street-level dealers in Australia found the main adulterants to be sugar, caffeine and paracetamol (Swift *et al.* 1999). Furthermore, heroin dealers interviewed in prison in the UK stated that the practice of 'cutting' heroin with dangerous adulterants was very infrequent (Coomber 1997). Finally, in a review of the aetiology of fatal heroin 'overdoses', Darke and Zador (1996) found little evidence to implicate contaminants in the causation of most of these fatalities.

Although patients occasionally report 'clots in the leg', the frequency of occurrence of a DVT after initiation of IOT is unknown. Concern about venous damage from injectable methadone is given as a reason by some patients for transfer to pharmaceutical heroin. However, it is not known whether injectable methadone does increase the risk of DVT more than injectable heroin. In the meantime the *Guidelines* advise that 'with the availability of injectable methadone there is very little clinical indication for prescribed diamorphine' (UK Department of Health 1999, p. 57). But what is the evidence for recommending injectable methadone ahead of injectable heroin?

The few data available (Metrebian *et al.* 1998; McCusker and Davies 1996; Hartnoll 1980) indicate that retention in heroin maintenance treatment is high and/or higher than in oral MMT. However, McCusker and Davies (1996) found that although more of their oral methadone sample dropped out of treatment, those who remained in oral MMT showed a reduction in prescribed opiate use and more were aiming at abstinence as a goal compared with the group prescribed heroin. These findings largely replicated those of Hartnoll *et al.* (1980).

Hartnoll *et al.* (1980), Battersby *et al.* (1992), McCusker and Davies (1996) and Metrebian *et al.* (1998) only examined outcomes of prescribed heroin between 6 and 12 months after initiation of treatment. Thorley *et al.* (1977), however, found that at a six-year follow-up of 128 patients prescribed heroin, only 23 per cent had remained continuously in treatment over this time period. More data are needed on long-term outcomes of both injectable heroin and methadone to assess whether patients are more likely to remain in IOT than transfer to oral MMT and/or become abstinent.

More data are also needed on the component(s) of the treatment package of IOT that accounts for its positive outcomes demonstrated in some studies. Edwards (1979) observes, 'it is far from certain that . . . the prescribing element in [IOT] considerably alters for the better the careers of a considerable proportion of addicts' (p. 9).

Until a consistent and substantial body of data is accumulated supporting sustained positive outcomes of IOT for both the individual patient *and the community*, the harm minimisation benefits of long-term IOT can only be speculative, however plausible the arguments may seem.

An ethical dilemma – is injectable opiate prescribing 'treatment'?

The above issues are central to the debate about whether maintenance on prescribed injectable opiates constitutes 'treatment'. Strang and Gossop (1994) noted the confusion between prescribing drugs as treatment and supplying drugs as commodities with the doctor being perceived as 'an overpaid grocer whose only task was to provide the products as requested . . .' (p. 202).

It is at this juncture that it is timely to pose the question, 'To what extent should "needle-fixation", i.e. the craving to inject, be accepted as a legitimate indication for prescription of injectable opiates?' How compatible is the medical maintenance of injecting drug behaviour with the ACMD's implication of injecting as a risk factor in drug-related deaths?

Some heroin users seek 'treatment' with injectable heroin for no other reason than to obtain legal supplies of heroin free of cost. Clearly there are benefits for these individuals that accrue from crime-free, cost-free heroin. The question is, are these benefits diminished if provided outside a paradigm of 'treatment'? That is, why not let social services (as an example) provide government supplies of heroin instead to those drug users uninterested in changing their heroin-using behaviour, and free-up places in drug treatment agencies for dependent users who do wish to cease or reduce injecting drugs?

Injectable opiate treatment raises other clinical and ethical issues. Is a prescriber obliged to train a patient to safely inject heroin or methadone into their femoral vein? What is a prescriber's legal liability in the event of a deep vein injecting related complication? What do harm minimisation principles imply should be the response to a patient seeking advice on safe injecting into the jugular vein because the femoral veins are no longer patent?

Should injectable opiate prescribing be a treatment option in Britain?

The *Guidelines* warn that commencing injectable prescribing may involve a long-term clinical commitment from both the patient and prescriber. In light of this caution, it is fascinating to contrast the commonly made objections to oral MMT by patients on the basis that it 'only prolongs the addiction' with the striking lack of objection made by the same patients to a prescription for injectable methadone. More research is required into heroin users' perceptions and beliefs about injectable and oral opiate maintenance treatment and their motivations for requesting either. More importantly, there is no information about how initial motives or goals of users entering IOT may change over time while in IOT.

It is not clear whether prescribers of IOT see themselves as providing indefinite maintenance or induction with a goal of eventual transfer to oral opiates. Furthermore, Sell *et al.* (1997) found that in a survey of 105 doctors (not all licensed) working in drug treatment prescribing services, less than half (49 per cent) of 35 licensed respondents thought that their patients had obtained a good clinical outcome with prescribed heroin.

Prescribers' ambivalence about heroin maintenance is further highlighted by Battersby *et al.* (1992) who found that no patient was given a heroin prescription unless they first requested it. Fear of being overwhelmed by demand for this intervention may have been a factor. However, Metrebian *et al.* (1998) did not support this perception when they found that not all patients sought a prescription for injectable heroin when offered a choice of it or injectable methadone – indeed one-third of subjects requested the latter.

So, 'decisions to prescribe heroin are often made for hypothetical, emotional or moral reasons or are based on clinical experience and personal belief rather than scientific evidence of effectiveness' (Metrebian *et al.* 1996, p. 196) – is this good clinical practice and is it sustainable?

How viable is the British model of injectable opiate prescribing?

It is timely to re-evaluate the practice of injectable heroin and methadone. The evidence to date clearly suggests there are benefits of prescribed heroin as implemented in Switzerland (Uchtenhagen 1997) and to a lesser degree in Britain, and scientific peer-refereed reports are expected soon from the Dutch heroin trials (only reported in press releases, internal reports and media coverage at the time of writing). But these benefits need to be better substantiated by more research. Britain has a unique opportunity to systematically describe and evaluate IOT because unlike most other countries, it already has heroin available as a licensed medication and has a treatment culture that tolerates prescription of injectable methadone.

It has been frequently reported that Britain's model of IOT is 'an endless source of fascination' to overseas observers. But of equal if not greater curiosity to the international field is Britain's paucity of evaluation of this intervention – all the more mystifying given its controversial status. Strang and Gossop (1994), McCusker and Davies (1996), Sell *et al.* (1997) and Metrebian *et al.* (1998) have all acknowledged the lack of scientific data and/or clinical protocol which underpins the practice of injectable opiate prescribing in this country. It would be easy to join the long line of these authors and finish this chapter with another clarion call for more research.

However, striving towards best practice in IOT depends on more than increasing the output of research evidence. The *Guidelines* advise 'in the absence of demonstrated significant superior outcomes from this form of clinical practice, and in recognition of the greater inherent dangers and the cost burden of such prescribing, services should regularly audit and review outcomes against set performance standards' (p. 55). Three decades ago, Edwards (1969) stated that 'the British system should indeed be seen in itself as an action experiment, and the results of that experiment should be *constantly monitored*, with a willingness, on the basis of research results, intelligently to change course' (p. 771).

It is puzzling to overseas researchers that a country that has consistently recognised the high level of international interest in this intervention cannot readily provide at any given point in time such fundamental data as number of patients prescribed IOT in Britain, the average dose of heroin or mean duration of treatment with injectable methadone. Elaborate randomised controlled trials are not required to, nor can they, generate this kind of information – attention to systematic data collection mechanisms by local treatment agencies will go a long way to improving clinical practice and consistency of treatment. Indeed the NHS's commitment to clinical governance and increased uniformity of treatment demands it.

Advocates of the British system argue its virtues to be a system of clinical freedom unfettered by regulatory requirements and national policy guidelines typical of other countries' drug treatment services. Therefore, demands to standardise the clinical practice of IOT is perceived by many as impinging on the liberty of individual doctors to practise as they see best for their patients. However this viewpoint places itself increasingly at odds with the sweeping changes being implemented by the NHS in its bid to raise the quality and consistency of health care in Britain.

The NHS, for example, is committed to ending the 'postcode' basis of access to best health care. However, as Sell *et al.* (1997) observed, 'provision of these treatments (injectable drugs including heroin and cocaine) is not based on research evidence nor on detailed policy regulations. The availability of the treatments varies widely with geographical location and depends on the personal opinion of specialists and on the willingness of local Health Commissions to pay for these services, which are several times more expensive than oral methadone treatment' (p. 222). The likelihood of a patient being prescribed injectable opiates may therefore depend more on the personal inclination of the medical practitioner than on the projected or identified needs of a community for access to IOT.

One could be provocative and call for the dissolution of the British system on the grounds that there is little evidence for its effectiveness as practised in Britain, that it is expensive to provide (compared with oral forms of maintenance treatment) and in so far as it is provided at all it is in an arbitrary and inequitable way by unaccountable clinicians, all attributes that violate recommended forms of good clinical practice in other areas of medicine in the UK.

However, too little is known about the benefits of IOT UK-style to demand its abolition either. Indeed, at the time of writing, expanded evaluated injectable heroin prescribing is being decisively considered by the government as one of a number of strategies to reduce crime in the country following the recommendations of the report of the House of Commons Select Committee on Home Affairs on the government's drugs policy (Home Affairs Committee 2002).

In conclusion, more rigorous systematic analysis and continuous quality improvement of IOT must be called forth. The modern paradigm of clinical governance expects it no less of 'the British system' than of any other form of medical practice in the UK.

References

Advisory Council on Misuse of Drugs (2000). Reducing drug related deaths. The Stationery Office, London.

Battersby, M., Farrell, M., Gossop, M., Robson, P. and Strang, J. (1992). 'Horse trading': prescribing injectable opiates to opiate addicts. A descriptive study. *Drug and Alcohol Review*, 11, 35–42.

Coomber, R. (1997). The adulteration of drugs: what dealers do to illicit drugs and what they think is done to them. *Addiction Research*, 5, 297–306.

Darke, S. and Zador, D. (1996). Fatal heroin 'overdose': a review. *Addiction*, 91, 1765–1772.

Darke, S., Hall, W., Weatherburn, D. and Lind, B. (1999). Fluctuations in heroin purity and the incidence of fatal heroin overdose. *Drug and Alcohol Dependence*, 54, 155–161.

Edwards, G. (1969). The British approach to the treatment of heroin addiction. *The Lancet*, i, 768–772.

Edwards, G. (1979). British policies on opiate addiction: ten years working of the revised response and options for the future. *British Journal of Psychiatry*, 134, 1–13.

Hall, W. (1999). Assessing the population-level impact of the Swiss model of heroin prescribing. Technical Report Number 76, National Drug and Alcohol Research Centre, Sydney.

Hartnoll, R. L., Mitcheson, M. C., Battersby, A., Brown, G., Ellis, M., Fleming, B. M. and Hedley, M. B. (1980). Evaluation of heroin maintenance in controlled trial. *Archives of General Psychiatry*, 37, 877–884.

House of Commons (2002). Home Affairs Select Committee. Hansard.

McCusker, C. and Davies, M. (1996). Prescribing drug of choice to illicit heroin users: the experience of a UK community drug team. *Journal of Substance Abuse Treatment*, 13, 521–531.

Metrebian, N., Shanahan, W. and Stimson, G. V. (1996). Heroin prescribing in the United Kingdom: an overview. *European Addiction Research*, 2, 194–200.

Metrebian, N., Shanahan, W., Wells, B. and Stimson, G. V. (1998). Feasibility of prescribing injectable heroin and methadone to opiate-dependent drug users: associated health gains and harm reductions. *Medical Journal of Australia*, 168, 596–600.

Metrebian, N., Carnwath, T., Stimson, G. and Storz, T. (2002). Survey of doctors prescribing diamorphine (heroin) to opiate-dependent drug users in the United Kingdom. *Addiction*, 97, 1155–1161.

Perneger, T. V., Giner, F., del Rio, M. and Mino, A. (1998). Randomised trial of heroin maintenance programme for addicts who fail in conventional drug treatments. *British Medical Journal*, 317, 13–18.

Powis, B., Strang, J., Griffiths, P., Taylor, C., Williamson, S., Fountain, J. and Gossop, M. (1999). Self-reported overdose among injecting drug users in London: extent and nature of the problem. *Addiction*, 94, 471–478.

Risser, D., Uhl, A., Stichenwirth, M., Honigschnabl, S., Hirz, W., Schneider, B., Stellwag-Carion, C., Klupp, N., Vycudilik, W. and Bauer, G. (2000). Quality of heroin and heroin-related deaths from 1987 to 1995 in Vienna, Austria. *Addiction*, 95, 375–382.

Sell, L., Farrell, M. and Robson, P. (1997). Prescription of diamorphine, dipipanone and cocaine in England and Wales. *Drug and Alcohol Review*, 16, 221–226.

Strang, J. and Gossop, M. (1994). *Heroin Addiction and Drug Policy: The British System*. Oxford University Press, Oxford.

Strang, J. and Sheridan, J. (1998). Effect of government recommendations on methadone prescribing in south east England: comparison of 1995 and 1997 surveys. *British Medical Journal*, 317, 1489–1490.

Strang, J. and Sheridan, J. (2002). Injectable methadone prescribing: a peculiarly British treatment. In Tober, G. and Strang, J. (eds) *Methadone Matters*. Dunitz, London.

Strang, J. and Sheridan, J. (2003). Effect of national guidelines on prescription of methadone: analysis of NHS prescription data, England 1990–2001. *British Medical Journal*, 327, 321–322.

Strang, J., Marsden, J., Cummins, M. *et al.* (2000). Randomised trial of supervised injectable versus oral methadone maintenance: report on feasibility and six-month outcome. *Addiction*, 95, 1631–1645.

Strang, J., Sheridan, J. and Barber, N. (1996). Prescribing injectable and oral methadone to opiate addicts: results from the 1995 national postal survey of community pharmacies in England and Wales. *British Medical Journal*, 313, 270–272.

Swift, W., Maher, L. and Dawson, M. (1999). Heroin purity and composition: an analysis of street-level samples in Cabramatta, New South Wales. Technical Report Number 79. National Drug and Alcohol Centre, Sydney.

Thorley, A., Oppenheimer, E. and Stimson, G. V. (1977). Clinic attendance and opiate prescription status of heroin addicts over a six-year period. *British Journal of Psychiatry*, 130, 565–569.

Uchtenhagen, A. (1997). Summary of the synthesis report. In Uchtenhagen, A., Gutzwiller, F. and Dobler-Mikola, A. (eds) *Programme for a Medical Prescription of Narcotics. Final Report of the Research Representatives* (pp. 1–11). Zurich Institute for Social and Preventive Medicine, University of Zurich.

UK Department of Health (1999). Drug misuse and dependence – guidelines on clinical management. The Stationery Office, London.

Chapter 11

Experimental amphetamine maintenance prescribing

Philip Fleming

Amphetamine misuse – a widespread but not a new problem

Amphetamine misuse is a world-wide phenomenon. The amphetamine-type stimulants (ATS) consist of two groups which share a basic chemical structure: the amphetamine and the ecstasy group. It has been estimated that 0.5 per cent of the world's population consume ATS which compares to figures of 0.14 per cent for opiates and 0.23 per cent for cocaine (World Drug Report 1997). The increasing sophistication of illicit manufacture and the greater profits from this production suggest that the problem of ATS abuse is likely to increase in the future.

In the United Kingdom there was early concern about the possible habit-forming properties of benzedrine – a form of amphetamine (Guttmann and Sargent 1937). But it was in the 1950s at a time when amphetamine was being quite widely prescribed for various conditions that concern was increasing about its misuse. In the 1960s widespread use of amphetamine amongst young people was first recognised (Connell 1965). This was mostly in the form of drinamyl, known as 'purple hearts' (a mixture of amphetamine and a barbiturate) and dexedrine, both of which came from the diversion of manufactured preparations, from chemist break-ins or as a result of excessive prescribing by doctors. In 1968 the excessive prescribing of injectable methamphetamine (methylamphetamine known as methedrine) by a small number of doctors led to an epidemic of the misuse of the drug (see below).

It has been the availability of illicitly manufactured amphetamine since the late 1970s that has led to the increase in amphetamine use in the past 20 years. Much of this increase occurred with little in the way of official statistics to note it. The Home Office Addicts Index did not record amphetamine users, though the problem was recognised by the Drugs Inspectorate. Bing Spear, the then Chief Inspector, commented in 1989: 'The abuse of amphetamine has continued to be a significant but largely unpublicised, and therefore not generally recognised, feature of the United Kingdom drug scene' (Standing Conference on Drug Abuse 1989: 1). The problem of injecting users only became apparent when the pilot needle exchange schemes were set up in 1987 when it was found that in some parts of the country injecting amphetamine users were accessing these services in significant numbers (Stimson *et al.* 1988).

Amphetamine is one of the United Kingdom's most commonly used illicit drug. Seizures of the drug have increased steadily, doubling between 1992 and 1994. A number of surveys have shown wide use of amphetamine by young people (Institute for the Study of Drug Dependence 1997). The most recent British Crime Survey figures show that 3 per cent of 16–19-year-olds have used amphetamine in the last year; this compares to 25 per cent who have used cannabis and 0.1 per cent who have used heroin (Condon and Smith, 2003). Many of these people, of course, only use the drug on a recreational basis. However, there are an increasing number of heavy dependent users many of whom inject the drug and who experience significant problems related to their drug use. The Department of Health Drug Misuse Statistics recorded data on users presenting to services based on the figures from the Regional Drug Misuse Databases. Overall, users presenting to agencies with amphetamine as their main drug of misuse formed 9 per cent of the total number and 11 per cent of those under age 20. There was considerable regional variation from 16 per cent in the South and West to 5 per cent in the Thames regions (Department of Health 1998). These figures do not necessarily reflect the true incidence of problematic amphetamine use as many users do not seek help for their problems.

The misuse of methamphetamine became a major problem in Japan in the late 1940s and the 1950s (Suwaki *et al.* 1997), partly following the appearance on the black market of army stocks left over from the war. Since the early 1970s there has been a further continuing epidemic of methamphetamine misuse from illicitly produced sources. Sweden experienced a significant amphetamine misuse problem in the 1950s and it continues to be a popular drug of misuse. Amongst injecting users it is the most frequently used drug (Kall 1997). In the United States amphetamine was increasingly prescribed for various conditions in the 1950s and this began to leak onto the black market in the 1960s. Around this time the first black market production of methamphetamine began and a surge in its use occurred particularly along the West Coast. Today there is evidence of resurgence in methamphetamine use in the USA. In recent years, ice, a smokable form of methamphetamine, has become a major problem in Hawaii (Klee 1997a). In Australia there was a small epidemic of amphetamine use in the late 1960s and early 1970s that lasted some years. Since the mid-1980s there has been a recurrence of epidemic amphetamine use that continues today. After cannabis, amphetamine is the most widely used illicit drug in Australia.

History of amphetamine prescribing – 1930s to 1960s

Amphetamine was first synthesised in 1887 and the related methamphetamine in 1919, but it was not before the 1930s that their therapeutic value was recognised. It was marketed as a nasal decongestant and was also used in the treatment of asthma and narcolepsy. Amphetamine and methamphetamine were widely prescribed to soldiers on both sides in World War II to combat fatigue, and during the 1940s and 1950s amphetamine was frequently prescribed as an aid to dieting and as a treatment for depression. There was increasing use too for occupational purposes: for example, amongst long-distance lorry drivers and others whose jobs required them to remain alert for long periods.

Problems associated with amphetamine were apparent relatively early, in particular misuse and increasing tolerance. In 1939 Benzedrine was put on Part 1 of the poisons list. In 1954 amphetamine-containing compounds – except for inhalers – became available only on prescription. As a result inhalers became a popular source of amphetamine. The 1964 Drugs (Prevention of Misuse Act) made the unauthorised possession of amphetamine-type drugs illegal.

The first experience of legal prescription of amphetamine for the treatment of addiction occurred in Sweden. Following pressure to liberalise drug policy, an experiment to prescribe central stimulants – principally oral amphetamine – and opiates by injection, for addicted persons commenced in April 1965 (Kall 1997). The aim was to provide unadulterated drugs, to reduce criminal activity, and after stabilisation to reduce the dosage and thereby cure the users of their addiction. The experiment was deemed a failure and was stopped in May 1967. It was the uncontrolled overgenerous prescribing of a single physician which led to significant leakage onto the black market and an increase in deaths of young people from overdoses that finally persuaded the authorities to discontinue such prescribing (Bejerot 1970).

In the summer of 1968 an epidemic of methamphetamine injecting occurred amongst young people in London, fuelled mainly by the excessive prescription of the drug by a few private doctors (Hawks et al. 1969). It came abruptly to an end in October of that year following the voluntary withdrawal by the manufacturers of supplies to retail pharmacists. Following the referral of a number of these users for help it was decided to take on a limited number and to prescribe methamphetamine in certain circumstances on a reducing basis. The total sample was of 23 patients with an average age of 20.8, most of whom in addition to daily methamphetamine injecting had a history of polydrug abuse. Twelve patients were prescribed methamphetamine. Only three of the total sample remained in contact after three months; two had come off all drugs and the third was making slow progress. This outcome was viewed somewhat pessimistically at the time, though it was concluded that 'there may be a place for very carefully considered prescribing' as part of the treatment response (Mitcheson et al. 1976).

An analysis of non-opioid users attending a drug dependence clinic in London in 1968/69 showed that half were young tablet users, 25 per cent of whom were receiving amphetamine prescriptions from GPs. The authors concluded that such 'maintenance prescribing' was unlikely to be effective, because of the widespread availability of illicit amphetamine (Gardner and Connell 1972).

Amphetamine prescribing – 1980s to date

As long ago as 1963 it was noted that the 'therapeutic indications for amphetamine prescription are to-day becoming vanishingly slight' (Oswald and Thacore 1963) and currently only narcolepsy and refractory hyper-kinetic states in children are cited as indications for its use (British National Formulary 1998).

The Misuse of Drugs Regulations 1985 places amphetamine under Schedule 2 and it can only be obtained by prescription. At the time of writing, any registered doctor can prescribe amphetamine. Hitherto, official advice has generally discouraged the prescription of amphetamine as a treatment for amphetamine misusers (Department of Health 1991; Advisory Council on the Misuse of Drugs 1993).

An increase in the amount of illicitly available amphetamine sulphate in the 1980s resulted in an increase in the number of problematic amphetamine misusers, though as explained above there was little in the way of official statistics to record this. A number of drug services in the UK had begun to see these problematic users and had to consider how best to help them. At a conference held by SCODA in 1989 several of these services reported their experiences (Standing Conference on Drug Abuse 1989). The preliminary results of an amphetamine prescribing service in Exeter were described, and the experience of the West Midlands Addiction Unit was reported. In both cases amphetamine prescribing was seen as a harm reduction strategy. In 1993 a conference held in Bristol heard reports of amphetamine prescribing from five services in Wales and South West England. Amphetamine was principally prescribed for injecting users with the aim of reducing injecting activity and the use of illicit amphetamine and of improving health status and reducing criminal activity. Although these were all open follow-up studies, improvements were found in the target behaviours; for example, all the studies showed a reduction in injecting behaviour (unpublished con-ference proceedings).

A more accurate indication of the extent of amphetamine prescribing in England and Wales was obtained in a survey of community pharmacies undertaken in 1995 (Strang and Sheridan 1997b). A one-in-four sample of pharmacies was sent a questionnaire and a 75 per cent response rate was achieved. Data was obtained on 177 amphetamine prescriptions dis-pensed which extrapolates to an estimated 900–1,000 patients receiving these prescriptions at any one time. This is approximately three times the number of addicts receiving a prescription of heroin (Strang and Sheridan 1997a). Considerable regional variation was found in the numbers of prescriptions of amphetamine dispensed. It was not clear whether this represented differences in the prevalence of amphetamine problems, or differences in the preference for the prescribing option in treatment.

A survey undertaken in 1996 reported on the attitudes and practice of senior doctors specialising in drug dependence in England and Wales in respect of substitute amphetamine prescribing (Bradbeer *et al.* 1998); 201 doctors were identified and a 74 per cent response was obtained. Overall 60 per cent of respondents saw a role for amphetamine prescribing whilst 46 per cent actually did so. Thirty-two per cent of respondents who did not prescribe amphetamine expressed an interest in doing so – lack of experience and budget restrictions being the main constraints. There was some variation between regions. The Thames regions had the lowest response rate (42 per cent), and the lowest percentage of those who saw a role for amphetamine prescribing. These services see fewer amphetamine users than those in other parts of the country (Department of Health 1998) and therefore have less experience of dealing with problematic users. The pressure to try alternative treatments has thus been less. Additionally the attitudes of senior doctors in the London clinics has been much more cautious with respect to such prescribing.

What is the rationale for prescribing amphetamine?

Most amphetamine users can be described as occasional recreational users. It is the smaller number of regular heavy amphetamine misusers who experience problems. Studies from many countries have demonstrated a wide range of serious harms arising from chronic amphetamine use. These include dependence, physical and psychological health problems as well as breakdown in social relationships (Klee 1992; Hall *et al.* 1993; Hando *et al.* 1997).

The issue of amphetamine dependence has been a contentious one as it has been argued that amphetamine substitution is inappropriate as users are not generally physically dependent. Measurable neurophysiological abnormalities were shown, in 1963, in six patients on their withdrawal from amphetamine-type stimulants (Oswald and Thacore 1963). The patients reported listlessness, depression and sleepiness in addition to craving. Other authors have described protracted symptoms of dysphoria, agitation and irritability, sleep disturbances, increased appetite and intense craving (Dackis and Gold 1990; Lago and Kosten 1994; Cantwell and McBride 1998). The broader concept of a dependence syndrome is now preferred as described in the Diagnostic and Statistical Manual of Mental Disorders, DSM-IV (American Psychiatric Association 1994). This emphasises the increased importance of amphetamine use over other activities, compulsion to use, amphetamine use becoming routine in the user's life, tolerance and the onset of withdrawal features. This has been shown to be valid in a study of amphetamine users (Topp and Darke 1997). A Severity of Amphetamine Dependence Questionnaire has been validated against DSM criteria and supports the existence of an amphetamine-dependence syndrome (Topp and Mattick 1997).

Many chronic amphetamine users inject the drug. Forty-five per cent of users presenting to services in England and Wales in the six months prior to September 1997 were injecting the drug (Department of Health 1998). A study in Edinburgh found that amphetamine was injected by more subjects (44 per cent) than any other drug with all the attendant risks of HIV and hepatitis C infection (Peters *et al.* 1997). In an Australian sample of regular amphetamine users two-thirds had injected the drug in the previous six months and 41 per cent had shared a needle in the previous month (Darke *et al.* 1994). Female amphetamine users engage in more high-risk sexual behaviour than heroin users (Klee 1997b). Other workers have described high levels of injecting among chronic amphetamine users presenting to drug clinics (see McBride *et al.* 1997; Charnaud and Griffiths 1998; Merrill and Tetlow 1998).

Amphetamine users often do not access treatment services as these services have historically been directed at opiate users (Klee 1992). A survey of stimulant users recruited from several different parts of England was undertaken to explore patterns of use and treatment needs in this group. They were much less likely to have received treatment for a stimulant problem than an opiate problem, and despite knowledge of services half said they would not seek help from a drug agency if they had problems with stimulants (Farrell *et al.* 1997).

Thus chronic amphetamine users are a group of people with a clear dependence syndrome who frequently inject the drug with associated physical and psychological morbidity and who infrequently access services. McBride looked at three areas in evaluating his amphetamine prescribing service: does it attract drug users; does it retain drug users in contact with the service; and does it change behaviour? The conclusion was that all three criteria had been met (McBride *et al.* 1997). Fleming and Roberts listed the following aims of their programme: to encourage users into the service; to reduce injecting and other behaviour; to reduce risk of spread of infections; to reduce illicit drug use; and to stabilise users' lifestyles (Fleming and Roberts 1994).

Mattick and Darke took a critical look at amphetamine substitution and listed the criteria that should be applied for the use of a drug in a maintenance programme: (i) regular frequent use (usually daily); (ii) clear evidence of dependence, preferably with neuro-adaptation; (iii) continued use having a severe effect on lifestyle; and (iv) the harms associated with 'street' use should be greater than those associated with replacement therapy. Generally they felt that these criteria were not met for most amphetamine users but conceded that 'maintenance may be appropriate to a minority of amphetamine

users' (Mattick and Darke 1995). Lintzeris *et al.* pointed out that the objectives of amphetamine substitution treatment are very similar to those of
methadone substitution; that is, the reduction of harms associated with the
individual's use of the drug. These included: reduction of illicit drug use;
reduction of transmission of blood-borne viruses; improving health and social
functioning; and the reduction of criminality associated with illicit drug use
(Lintzeris *et al.* 1996).

Potential harms associated with amphetamine prescribing

Possible harms are mentioned by a number of authors. These include toxic
effects, adverse effects on mental health including the precipitation of psychotic episodes, and neurotoxic effects (Fleming and Roberts 1994; Mattick
and Darke 1995; Merrill and Tetlow 1998).

Toxic effects have been reported from both acute and chronic use and
there have been reports of death occurring (Derlet *et al.* 1989). However,
such deaths are rare and are usually associated with cardiovascular events
such as cerebrovascular accident or cardiac arrest.

The adverse mental health effects of amphetamine were first brought
into prominence by Connell who described a psychotic illness often indistin-
guishable from schizophrenia in amphetamine users (Connell 1958). Hawks
et al. reported a high proportion of their cohort of methamphetamine users
experienced delusions and hallucinations (Hawks *et al.* 1976). Hall *et al.*
found psychological morbidity was common in their series of amphetamine
misusers. The most common symptoms were: depression (79 per cent), anxiety
(76 per cent), paranoia (52 per cent) and hallucinations (46 per cent). Those
users with a history of psychotic illness are particularly vulnerable to relapse
which may be precipitated by amphetamine use (Hall *et al.* 1996).

The issue of neurotoxic effects is a complex one. The amphetamine group
of drugs has effects on several neurotransmitter systems including cate-
cholamine, dopaminergic, noradrenaline and 5-HT (Holman 1994). Animal
studies have shown that chronic exposure to amphetamine can cause depletion
of these neurotransmitters (Gawin and Ellinwood 1988; Ricaurte *et al.* 1991;
Grace 1995). The relevance of this to drug misusers is not clear. A recent
study showed evidence of a reduction of brain 5-HT in MDMA users, though
whether these changes are reversible or permanent is not clear. Neither is it
clear what functional consequences may follow such 5-HT depletion (McCann
et al. 1998).

Amphetamine programme characteristics

The main considerations in prescribing amphetamine have been summarised:
(Fleming 1998) based on survey data; (Strang and Sheridan 1997b; Bradbeer

et al. 1998) on information directly from a number of prescribers; and reports of prescribing programmes (McBride *et al.* 1997; Charnaud and Griffiths 1998; Merrill and Tetlow 1998). Prescribing should be part of a treatment package that includes appropriate counselling and support and help with any medical, social or family problems.

Indications

Primary amphetamine users with heavy problematic use. This is normally daily use of over 1 gram of street amphetamine a day, or on most days a week. In practice heavy users may take several grams a day and will have been using amphetamine regularly for several months. Services mostly prescribe for injecting users though some will consider prescribing for heavy non-injecting users.

Contra-indications

These include a history of mental illness (particularly psychosis), hypertension, heart disease or pregnancy.

Dosage and form

Calculating dosage is not always easy as street amphetamine varies in purity. Though mostly of low purity (5 per cent), higher purity 'paste' is increasingly common in the UK (Forensic Science Service – personal communication). Some prescribers attempt to match street dosages, others aim to minimise craving and withdrawal symptoms. The survey of community pharmacies (Strang and Sheridan 1997b) found a mean upper dose for oral amphetamine of 41 mg daily. The survey of prescribers found a mean upper limit of 66 mg (Bradbeer *et al.* 1998). Many practitioners have an upper limit of 60 mg, although some prescribed higher doses, e.g. 80–100 mg in some cases.

Amphetamine has a variable half-life depending on the pH of the urine (Rowland 1969); the average is about twelve hours. Some practitioners alkalinise the urine to increase the half-life (Sherman 1990). Once-a-day dosing is sufficient, though sometimes divided doses are given.

Currently more prescriptions are in the form of tablets than of oral liquid preparations. The survey of prescribers found 57 per cent tablets, 21 per cent liquid and 2 per cent ampoules, which was similar to the pharmacy survey: 73 per cent tablets, 23 per cent liquid and 3 per cent ampoules. There is little evidence of injecting of oral preparations whether in the form of liquid or tablets. It is easier to supervise the consumption of a liquid preparation and this is likely to be less attractive on the black market than tablets.

Monitoring

This usually includes: assessment of mental state; inspection of injection sites; monitoring of physical state including blood pressure and weight; and urinalysis for the presence of other drugs. Recently a technique has been described that will allow the distinction between prescribed and street amphetamine in urine samples (Tetlow and Merrill 1996). This allows the more accurate assessment of any continuing illicit amphetamine use.

How long should prescribing continue?

There is little research to guide practitioners and as a result there are differing views. Some argue that if patients are showing benefit from a prescription and they relapse if this is discontinued the balance of advantage lies in continuing the prescription. Others argue whilst the long-term effects on the brain of prescribing amphetamine are unclear, such prescribing should be time-limited.

Is amphetamine prescribing an effective intervention?

Until recently there has been little research on the treatment of problematic amphetamine use (Klee 1992) and particularly a lack of controlled studies (Mattick 1994; Mattick and Darke 1995).

There is only one case control study (Klee 1995). Clients presenting to drug treatment agencies in north west England with amphetamine problems were matched with controls recruited through community agencies, and followed-up over six to eight months. Users were daily or very frequent users and 59 per cent were injecting. Forty-three per cent were prescribed amphetamine. The dose levels varied and were adjusted and monitored by the treating physicians. The main findings were that the use of street drugs and the frequency of injecting was less in the prescribed group in comparison to the control group. Psychological health was poor in the early months and improved in those receiving counselling. Those prescribed amphetamine were less likely than controls to persist in criminal activities.

McBride and colleagues reported on a group of 63 clients who had received prescriptions of amphetamine (McBride *et al.* 1997). These were compared with 25 clients who met the same criteria but who had attended the service before amphetamine prescribing began. The inclusion criteria included having a primary amphetamine problem and the injection of amphetamine in the week before the assessment interview. There were significant increases in the number and proportion of amphetamine users attending the service and in the duration of contact with the treatment group. There were reductions in the quantity and frequency of illicit amphetamine use, in injecting and in needle sharing among the treatment group. McBride notes the methodological weaknesses of the study and states the conclusions should be interpreted with caution.

Charnaud and Griffiths, in a retrospective case note study, compared clients discharged from treatment during 1995 and 1996 who had been pre-scribed either oral methadone or oral dexamphetamine (Charnaud and Griffiths 1998). All had been intravenous drug users who had been injecting on a daily basis for a minimum of six months prior to referral. Levels of injecting drug use had reduced to a similar extent in both groups with 67 per cent of the opiate users and 70 per cent of the amphetamine misusers having stopped injecting.

In a prospective study, Merrill followed up amphetamine users who were prescribed oral dexamphetamine in a structured programme, for a period of twelve months (Merrill and Tetlow 1998). Criteria for prescribing included using at least 1 gm of street amphetamine on at least four days a week; 66 per cent were injecting the drug. Merrill used a urine screening test that could distinguish between street and prescribed amphetamine (Tetlow and Merrill 1996). The use of illicit amphetamine fell substantially as did the frequency of injecting – most of these improvements occurred early in treatment. Over the twelve-month period there was a significant improvement in psychological health as measured by the GHQ scores. In a retrospective study Fleming and Roberts reviewed the first three years' operation of a closely monitored amphetamine prescribing programme (Fleming and Roberts 1994). Inclusion criteria were six months daily inject-ing of amphetamine in primary users of the drug. The major improvement was seen in injecting activity which decreased in all subjects and ceased in over half.

Many of the studies quoted have methodological limitations and only one is case controlled. Nevertheless there are similarities in the results. All show a reduction in injecting activity in clients prescribed amphetamine. Improvements in psychological functioning were reported. There is a reduction in reported street amphetamine use and this was confirmed in the one study that discriminated illicit from prescribed amphetamine in urine testing. Reduction in criminal activity is reported in some studies. The attraction and retention in treatment of problematic amphetamine users is improved. It is interesting to note that these are exactly the same ben-efits that come from oral methadone treatment for opiate users (Farrell *et al.* 1994).

What of adverse effects of amphetamine prescribing? In the studies quoted, subjects were psychiatrically screened and episodes of paranoid sympto-matology rarely followed amphetamine prescription. It is not possible from the data available to draw any conclusions about any adverse effects of long-term amphetamine ingestion. Although most subjects had been using amphetamine heavily for many months before treatment, the length of treatment was usually less than two years.

Conclusion

Clinical studies suggest that there are benefits to be obtained from the prescription of oral amphetamine, in particular to heavily dependent intravenous amphetamine users. These benefits are in the reduction of harms to the drug user. Amphetamine prescribing should be done in the context of carefully structured programmes, and subjects should be carefully screened and monitored. Little in the way of ill effects has been reported. The evidence base for such prescribing is still relatively weak and there is a need for more in the way of controlled studies (Mattick and Darke 1995; Lintzeris *et al.* 1996).

References

Advisory Council on the Misuse of Drugs (1993). AIDS and drug misuse update report. London: HMSO.

American Psychiatric Association (1994). *Diagnostic and Statistical Manual of Mental Disorders* (Fourth Edition) Washington, D.C.: American Psychiatric Association.

Bejerot, N. (1970). The years of chaos in Swedish drug policy. Chapter 7. *Addiction and Society*, Springfield, Illinois: Charles Thomas.

Bradbeer, T. M., Fleming, P. M., Charlton, P. and Crichton, J. S. (1998). Survey of amphetamine prescribing in England and Wales. *Drug and Alcohol Review* 17, 299–304.

British National Formulary (1998). British Medical Association and the Royal Pharmaceutical Society of Great Britain.

Cantwell, B. and McBride, A. J. (1998). Self detoxification by amphetamine dependent patients: a pilot study. *Drug and Alcohol Dependence* 49, 157–163.

Charnaud, B. and Griffiths, V. (1998). Levels of intravenous drug misuse among clients prescribed oral dexamphetamine or oral methadone: a comparison. *Drug and Alcohol Dependence* 52, 79–84.

Condon, J. and Smith N. (2003). Prevalence of drug use: Key findings from the 2002/2003 British Crime Survey. London: Home Office.

Connell, P. H. (1958). Amphetamine Psychosis. Maudsley Monograph Number 5, Institute of Psychiatry. London: Oxford University Press.

Connell, P. H. (1965). Adolescent drug taking. *Proceedings of the Royal Society for Medicine* 58, 409–412.

Dackis, C. A. and Gold, M. S. (1990). Addictiveness of central stimulants. *Advances in Alcohol and Substance Abuse* 9, 9–26.

Darke, S., Cohen, J., Ross, J., Hando, J. and Hall, W. (1994). Transitions between routes of administration of regular amphetamine users. *Addiction* 89, 1077–1083.

Department of Health (1991). Drug Misuse and Dependence: Guidelines on Clinical Management. London: HMSO.

Department of Health (1998). Drug Misuse Statistics 1997. London: Department of Health.

Derlet, R. W., Rice, P., Horowitz, Z. and Lord, R. V. (1989). Amphetamine toxicity: experience with 127 cases. *Journal of Emergency Medicine* 7, 157–161.

Farrell, M., Ward, J., Mattick, R., Hall, W., Stimson, G. V., des Jarlais, D., Gossop, M. and Strang, J. (1994). Methadone maintenance treatment in opiate dependence: a review. *British Medical Journal* 309, 997–1001.

Farrell, M., Howes, S., Griffiths, P., Williamson, S., Bacchus, L. and Taylor, C. (1997). Stimulant Needs Assessment Project. Report to the Department of Health. National Addiction Centre, London.

Fleming, P. M. (1998). Prescribing amphetamine to amphetamine users as a harm reduction measure. *International Journal of Drug Policy* 9, 399–344.

Fleming, P. M. and Roberts, D. (1994). Is the prescription of amphetamine justified as a harm reduction measure? *Journal of the Royal Society of Health* 114, 127–131.

Gardner, R. and Connell, P. H. (1972). Amphetamine and other non-opioid drug users attending a Special Drug Dependence Clinic. *British Medical Journal* 2, 322–325.

Gawin, F. H. and Ellinwood, E. H. (1988). Cocaine and other stimulants: actions, abuse and treatment. *New England Journal of Medicine* 318, 18, 1173–1182.

Grace, A. A. (1995). The tonic/phasic model of dopamine system regulation: its relevance for understanding how stimulant abuse can alter basal ganglia function. *Drug and Alcohol Dependence* 37, 111–129.

Guttmann, E. and Sargent, W. (1939). Observations on benzedrine. *British Medical Journal* 1, 1013.

Hall, W., Darke, S., Ross, M. and Wodak, A. (1993). Patterns of drug use and risk-taking among injecting amphetamine and opioid drug users in Sydney, Australia. *Addiction* 88, 509–516.

Hall, W., Hando, J., Darke, S. and Ross, J. (1996). Psychological morbidity and route of administration among amphetamine users in Sydney, Australia. *Addiction* 91, 81–17.

Hando, J., Topp, L. and Hall, W. (1997). Amphetamine-related harms and treatment preferences of regular amphetamine users in Sydney, Australia. *Drug and Alcohol Dependence* 46, 105–113.

Hawks, D., Mitcheson, M., Ogborne, A. and Edwards, G. (1969). Abuse of methylamphetamine. *British Medical Journal* 2, 715–721.

Holman, R. B. (1994). Biological effects of central nervous system stimulants. *Addiction* 89, 1435–1441.

Institute for the Study of Drug Dependence (1997). *Drug Misuse in Britain 1996.* London: Institute for the Study of Drug Dependence.

Kall, K. (1997). Amphetamine abuse in Sweden. In *Amphetamine Misuse: International Perspectives on Current Trends*, ed. Klee, H. Amsterdam: Harwood Academic Publishers.

Klee, H. (1992). A new target for behavioural research – amphetamine misuse. *British Journal of Addiction* 87, 439–446.

Klee, H. (1995). *Amphetamine Misuse and Treatment: An Exploration of Individual and Policy Impediments to Effective Service Delivery*. Manchester: Manchester Metropolitan University.

Klee, H. (ed.) (1997a). *Amphetamine Misuse: International Perspectives on Current Trends*. Amsterdam: Harwood Academic Publishers.

Klee, H. (1997b). Amphetamine injecting women and their primary partners: an analysis of risk behaviour. In *The Impact of AIDS. Psychological and Social Aspects of HIV Infection*, eds Catalan, J., Sherr, L. and Hodge, B. Amsterdam: Harwood Academic Publishers.

Lago, J. and Kosten, T. R. (1994). Stimulant withdrawal. *Addiction* 89, 1477–1481.

Lintzeris, N., Holgate, F. and Dunlop, D. (1996). Addressing dependent amphetamine use: a place for prescription. *Drug and Alcohol Review* 15, 189–195.

McBride, A. J., Sullivan, G., Blewett, A. E. and Morgan, S. (1997). Amphetamine prescribing as a harm reduction measure: a preliminary study. *Addiction Research* 5, 95–112.

McCann, U. D., Szabo, Scheffel, U., Dannals, R. F. and Ricaurte, G. A. (1998). Positron emission tomographic evidence of toxic effect of MDMA ('Ecstasy') on brain serotonin neurons in human beings. *Lancet* 352, 1433–1437.

Mattick, R. P. (1994). Maintenance approaches to treating drug misusers: a review of the empirical evidence. National Drug and Alcohol Research Centre, University of New South Wales, Sydney, Australia.

Mattick, R. P. and Darke, S. (1995). Drug replacement treatments: is amphetamine substitution a horse of a different colour? *Drug and Alcohol Review* 14, 389–394.

Merrill, J. and Tetlow, T. (1998). Prescribing for amphetamine users: evaluation of a dexamphetamine substitution programme. Paper presented at the First National Conference on Stimulants. Manchester Metropolitan University, 18 September 1998.

Mitcheson, M., Edwards, G., Hawks, D. and Ogbourne, A. (1976). Treatment of methylamphetamine users during the 1968 epidemic. In Edwards, G., Russell, M. A. H., Hawks, A. and MacCafferty, M. (eds) *Drugs and Drug Dependence*, London: Saxon House Publishers.

Oswald, I. and Thacore, V. R. (1963). Amphetamine and phenmetrazine addiction: physiological abnormalities in the abstinence syndrome. *British Medical Journal* 427–431.

Peters, A., Davies, T. and Richardson, A. (1997). Increasing popularity of injection as the route of administration of amphetamine in Edinburgh. *Drug and Alcohol Dependence* 48, 227–234.

Ricaurte, G. A., Martello, M. B., Wilson, M. A., Molliver, M. E., Katz, J. L. and Martello, A. L. (1991). Dexfenfluramine neurotoxicity in brains of non-human primates. *Lancet* 338, 1487–1488.

Rowland, M. (1969). Amphetamine blood and urine levels in man. *Journal of Pharmaceutical Science* 58, 508–509.

Sherman, J. P. (1990). Dexamphetamine for 'speed' addiction. *Medical Journal of Australia* 153, 306.

Standing Conference on Drug Abuse (1989). Working with Stimulant Users: Report of SCODA Conference held on 5 October 1989. London: Standing Conference on Drug Abuse.

Stimson, G. V., Alldritt, Dolan, K., Donoghoe, M. and Lart, R. (1988). Injecting equipment exchange schemes. Final Report. London: Goldsmiths' College.

Strang, J. and Sheridan, J. (1997a). Heroin-prescribing in the 'British System' of the mid 1990s: data from the national survey of community pharmacies in England and Wales. *Drug and Alcohol Review* 16, 7–16.

Strang, J. and Sheridan, J. (1997b). Prescribing amphetamines to drug misusers: data from the 1995 national survey of community pharmacies in England and Wales. *Addiction* 92, 833–838.

Suwaki, H., Fukui, S. and Konuma, K. (1997). Methamphetamine abuse in Japan: its 45 year history and the current situation. In *Amphetamine Misuse: International Perspectives on Current Trends*, ed. Klee, H. Amsterdam: Harwood Academic Publishers.

Tetlow, V. A. and Merrill, J. (1996). Rapid determination of amphetamine stereo-isomer ratios in urine by gas chromatography–mass spectroscopy. *Annals of Clinical Biochemistry* 33, 50–54.

Topp, L. and Darke, S. (1997). The applicability of the dependence syndrome to amphetamine. *Drug and Alcohol Dependence* 48, 113–118.

Topp, L. and Mattick, R. P. (1997). Validation of the amphetamine dependence syndrome and the SamDQ. *Addiction* 92, 151–162.

World Drug Report (1997). *United Nations International Drug Control Programme*. Oxford: Oxford University Press.

Chapter 12

Needle exchange in Britain

Janie Sheridan

Introduction

The distribution of sterile injecting equipment and somewhere to dispose safely of used equipment, in the form of needle exchange schemes, has become a part of the harm reduction approach to managing problem drug use in Great Britain. The availability of sterile injecting equipment underpins many of the other harm minimisation measures in place such as advice on how to inject safely, not to share needles and syringes and other paraphernalia, and the ease with which different viruses may be transmitted.

Early policy interventions such as the provision of needle exchange and harm minimisation messages, expansion of methadone programmes, major changes in the philosophy surrounding the management of drug misuse from an abstinence orientation to a harm reduction response, are all considered to have contributed to the low levels of HIV currently seen in the UK. As Gerry Stimson concluded, 'The UK experience adds to the growing evidence of the significance of early interventions in encouraging behaviour change (of injecting drug users) and limiting the spread of HIV . . .' (Stimson 1995, p. 713). While the success of preventing an HIV epidemic cannot be attributed solely to needle exchange, it has undoubtedly had a huge impact on the incidence of new HIV infections. Other measures such as health education messages, government media campaigns and access to treatment have all played their part.

This, of course, was not always the case. As details of HIV and AIDS began to emerge, the UK and other countries began to fear an epidemic. Policy was slow to develop at first. Berridge and Strong describe three stages of 'AIDS policy' in the UK: the construction of a policy community (1981–1986) starting at a local level, with gay activists and clinical experts working together to form a 'policy community' dealing with the Government's interest in public health; a period of 'wartime emergency' (1986–1987), during which time the Government embraced AIDS as a political priority, and a stage of normalisation from 1988 onwards where HIV has become a part of normal policy responses (Berridge and Strong 1991). It was during the 'wartime emergency period' that the supply of clean injecting equipment in the form of needle exchange started in the UK. Such a potentially revolutionary policy was a typical result of such a period of policy change.

Needle exchange is not specific to the UK, and exists in many other countries. The common aim is to distribute sterile injecting equipment and to provide a safe place for used equipment to be disposed, in order to minimise the transmission of blood-borne viruses such as HIV and hepatitis B and C. However, policy and practice vary. For example, in New Zealand, clients pay a nominal sum for their equipment. In some parts of Europe, an exchange is strictly on a one-for-one basis. In a UK context, needle exchange is 'a facility where drug injectors can obtain sterile needles and syringes in return for used injecting equipment. It is free to the client, and available on a regular reliable basis at a known location' (Donoghoe *et al.* 1992). Syringe exchanges operate from drug agencies, drug treatment clinics, accident and emergency departments, mobile units, voluntary agencies, outreach services and community pharmacies.

The syringe as an instrument of drug administration

Christopher Wren, in the 1650s, administered opium to a dog using a quill and small bladder (Macht 1916). Others experimented with injecting into human veins during the seventeenth century and it is reported that one of the first drugs used was opium (Macht 1916). After this time, injecting was mainly used for introducing chemicals into corpses to aid examination, but a revival of intravenous injecting into live humans occurred at the end of the eighteenth century.

The spread of the popularity of injecting opiates may be attributed to two factors – the effectiveness of opiates as analgesics and the speed of onset of action through the injecting route. Nowadays, injecting is not simply limited to opiates, and the problems associated with injecting relate both to the drug itself and to the route of administration. Whilst needle exchange was primarily concerned with preventing the spread of HIV, we shall see that it has expanded its remit to cover aspects of safer injecting practices, general advice on health, the prevention of spread of other viruses such as hepatitis B and C, safer sex and to act as a potential gateway into treatment.

Sharing of injecting equipment

The use of contaminated injecting equipment was recognised as one way in which HIV could be transmitted. In Edinburgh, Dr Roy Robertson examined samples of blood taken from his injecting drug-using patients and found an HIV rate of 51 per cent. The lack of available sterile injecting equipment was thought to be in part to blame for this situation (Robertson *et al.* 1986), resulting in drug users reusing and sharing needles and syringes. Roy

Robertson describes how, early in the 1980s, injectors rented used injecting equipment, often contaminated with blood. This lack of injecting equipment was further compounded with a restriction on pharmacists selling needles and syringes and police activity to reduce the availability of injecting equipment (see Chapter 10, Volume I, by Roy Robertson). This outbreak did not become a widespread epidemic across the UK.

Sharing may take place between individuals on many levels – between sexual partners, between friends, between drug users in the same community. McKeganey and Barnard noted a number of influences on the decision to share including the availability of injecting equipment, the immediate need to inject, assessments of risk – for example, injectors may consider family and friends to be 'safe' whilst strangers are considered less safe, and social context – for example, it may be difficult to refuse to give used equipment to a close friend without insulting them (McKeganey and Barnard 1992).

An important distinction must also be made between lending and borrowing. There is no risk of the lender contracting blood-borne viruses if the lender used clean equipment and does not re-use the lent equipment, but there is a high risk of transmission for the borrower (McKeganey and Barnard 1992).

Supplying clean injecting equipment prior to needle exchange

An uneasy situation had existed prior to the early 1980s in community pharmacies in England and Wales with regard to the sales of clean injecting equipment. While pharmacists were not prohibited from selling syringes to injecting drug users, there was often a reluctance on the part of pharmacists to supply. Injectors would therefore employ a number of tactics in order to obtain syringes such as claiming that they, or a relative, were diabetic.

In 1982, the Royal Pharmaceutical Society of Great Britain (RPSGB), the professional body for pharmacy in Great Britain, became concerned with the supply of needles and syringes for injecting drug users by community pharmacists and decided on a prohibition of this activity (RPSGB 1982). However, in 1986, with the growing emergence of concerns relating to HIV, the RPSGB issued a statement allowing community pharmacists to supply clean injecting equipment to injecting drug users (RPSGB 1986). This reversal of previous advice paved the way for pharmacists to become major players in the supply of injecting equipment to injecting drug users including their eventual inclusion in needle exchange schemes following the Government pilot needle exchange study in 1987 (see later).

In Scotland, the situation was complicated further due to the common law crime of 'reckless behaviour' which could criminalise the act of selling injecting equipment for use with illicit drugs. However, the Lord Advocate has since stated that prosecutions would not take place against 'Designated officers' or staff at needle exchanges who provide needles and syringes in the context of needle exchange.

In the 1980s in Amsterdam, it was concerns over the spread of hepatitis B which led to the setting up of a needle exchange service. Local community pharmacies provided all the clean injecting equipment to injecting drug users. However, due to overwhelming demand, the pharmacies decided they could no longer provide this service. The *junkiebond* approached the local government health department and arranged for them to distribute clean injecting equipment via the *junkiebond*, and also to provide for a place for safe disposal, leading to the birth of a needle exchange service. By 1989, around 800,000 needles and syringes had been distributed by 11 exchange facilities including the methadone bus (Hartgers *et al.* 1989). A returns rate of 70 per cent was increased to over 80 per cent once a policy of one-for-one had been instigated (Rezza *et al.* 1994).

A typically British response...

The emergence of HIV caused a change in the way the medical profession focused on disease. Historically, public health measures and vaccination programmes had been hugely successful in eradicating diseases such as bubonic plague, cholera and polio, and this resulted in a certain degree of smugness and complacency. With the emergence, however, of an untreatable, fatal infection a sense of security regarding western medicine's ability to deal with any infection was shattered.

Initially, the Government was slow to respond to the threat of HIV, leaving much of the work to Sir Donald Acheson, the Chief Medical Officer at the time. He found himself battling against Government apathy.

It was not until 1986 that the government really embraced the notion of HIV as an 'epidemic' and in response to the threat of the virus spreading rapidly through the injecting drug-user community, and the potential for further spread into the rest of the community through sexual contact between injecting and non-injecting individuals, a rapid investigation into the distribution of sterile injecting equipment commenced.

The setting up of the needle exchange schemes

The emergence of HIV and its rapid spread through certain communities overseas caused the Government to start to formulate policies to prevent this, including some more innovative and less acceptable, and therefore braver, responses such as the provision of free needles and syringes to injecting drug users. However, it appeared that the setting up of needle exchange programmes was relatively unopposed by the public in England and this could be in part due to the general public being made aware of the risks of contracting HIV through injecting equipment through the major Government education campaign of the 1980s, which focused on changes in sexual behaviour and the risks of injecting drugs with shared equipment (Day and Klein 1990). This public education campaign has been considered to be 'the initiative which distinguishes the British policy response from that of other countries' (Day and Klein 1990).

The discussions about the provision of sterile injecting equipment had at least some echo of the discussions about the provision of medical treatment to addicts, sixty years before. The 1926 Rolleston Report into opiate addiction concluded that there should be 'legitimate and medical treatment with morphine and heroin, for those who required gradual withdrawal and also those incapable of withdrawal or whose social habits deteriorated when not supplied with regular allowances of the drug'. Some have argued that there were, within this confirmation of the medical 'ownership' of opiate addiction, elements of a harm minimisation philosophy similar to that which surrounds the provision of sterile injecting equipment to individuals who are unable or unwilling to stop injecting drugs.

The needle exchange pilot

Needle exchange schemes were established as local initiatives during 1986 in various parts of the country, but without any 'official' position on their suitability (or otherwise). Urgent internal discussions occurred between the Government health officials and their advisers about whether these schemes were mistaken developments and should be closed down, or were pioneering new developments that should be embraced and promoted (John Strang, personal communication). In the event, the chosen path was somewhere in between. The Department of Health and Social Security and the Scottish Home and Health Department decided to give cautious support, but support nevertheless, and to announce an official pilot needle exchange initiative. And so, in 1987, 15 pilot schemes were selected as being the cohort of newly-created needle-and-syringe exchange schemes (including the few recently-established needle exchanges which already existed in some parts of the country prior to this initiative), and with an evaluation (to be conducted by Gerry Stimson) commencing in April 1987. The decision was considered to be controversial, especially as some countries such as the USA were deciding to restrict the supply of clean injecting equipment. There were four main requirements of the schemes:

- to provide equipment on an exchange basis;
- to provide assessment and/or counselling on clients' drug problems;
- to provide advice on safer sex and offer HIV test counselling; and
- to collect data for the pilot evaluation.

In Stimson's evaluation of the pilot, it was concluded that the programme had been satisfactorily set up, and had reached injecting drug users in considerable numbers (769 clients between June and October 1987), but there was a large turnover of clients. Many of these clients were found not to be in touch with other drug agencies. The main reasons stated for users attending the services were a concern about AIDS and a lack of clean injecting equipment (Stimson *et al.*, 1988).

After the pilot

The Government's Advisory Council on the Misuse of Drugs presented its first report on AIDS and Drug Misuse in 1988. The report recommended an expansion of needle exchange schemes and further harm minimisation measures. There were some concerns in government about some of the measures recommended, delaying the publication of the report until early 1988 (Berridge and Strong 1991).

There followed a rapid expansion in needle exchange schemes rising to over 200 needle exchange schemes in England, Wales and Scotland by 1990 (Dolan *et al.* 1993). They operated from a number of environments such as drug treatment clinics, community drug teams, voluntary street agencies, outreach and through community pharmacies. A range of equipment was offered, including a choice of syringes, swabs, condoms, sterile water, bleach and dressings, despite a quirk in UK law, which at the time rendered supplying any 'paraphernalia', apart from needles and syringes, illegal. Additional services offered were advice and referral with regard to drug use, HIV and safer-sex counselling, primary health care, legal and housing advice and substitute prescribing.

Not all services provided all the above and the 1989 national survey of syringe exchanges in England noted a lack of central co-ordination and supervision among schemes, thus allowing for services to be sensitive to local needs (Lart and Stimson 1990). Of the 55 schemes which responded to this study, 42 were based in drug agencies, eight in pharmacies, two 'stand-alone' and the remainder in other health-related agencies. They were split between the NHS and voluntary sector. In addition to the variety of service bases, the non-pharmacy scheme staff backgrounds also varied, including registered mental nurses, registered general nurses, health visitors and those who describe themselves as 'drug workers'. Within pharmacy schemes, the issuing of equipment was most often carried out by pharmacy staff, even though the RPSGB has recommended that this be done by a qualified pharmacist (Council of the RPSGB 1993). Although more accessible, pharmacy schemes offered limited services compared to drug agency schemes.

Pharmacy needle exchanges

While in no way specific to the UK, community pharmacy in Britain has embraced an involvement in harm reduction activities. A 1995 national survey of community pharmacies in England and Wales found 19 per cent of responding pharmacies involved in needle exchange, and 35 per cent currently selling sterile injecting equipment not as part of a needle exchange service (Sheridan *et al.* 1996). Pharmacists report few serious problems relating to service provision, although theft from the pharmacy and intoxicated clients are more common occurrences (Sheridan *et al.* 2000).

Pharmacy needle exchange differs from other exchange services in that it takes place in the context of a retail environment, where other non-drug-using members of the public will be accessing health care. Those providing this service are not normally specialists in drug misuse and in many cases are willing to offer only a simple exchange service and limited advice and referral facilities. Other operational factors such as lack of privacy also limit the availability of other services such as advice on HIV testing and safer sex. However, some pharmacists have become very proactive in providing services for injecting drug users offering needle exchange, dispensing methadone prescriptions, supervising the consumption of methadone in the pharmacy and liaising closely with other agencies.

Pharmacy-based schemes are generally open longer hours than non-pharmacy schemes (Lart and Stimson 1990), and were found to offer needle exchange for a mean of 55 hours per week in services offered in the South East of England (Sheridan *et al.* 2000). Clients of these services rated the location, opening hours and approachability of staff as good, but many suggested improving the range of equipment on offer and publicity for such schemes (Parson *et al.*, 2000). In comparison, non-pharmacy needle exchange services provide additional services such as primary health care, counselling on HIV, hepatitis testing and referral into treatment, although they may have more restricted opening hours and be sited in less convenient locations.

But it encourages injecting, doesn't it?

Needle exchange has had many opponents – major concerns have been that there would be an increase in drug use, a perceived condoning of injecting drug use and an increase in used injecting equipment left in community areas near to needle exchanges. Research from abroad has indicated that the availability of free injecting equipment does not increase the frequency of injecting drug use (Wolk *et al.* 1990). A preliminary study in San Francisco noted that there was no increase in injecting drug use, no increase in sharing of injecting equipment or a shift to injecting (Guydish *et al.* 1993). The introduction of needle exchange has also been shown not to encourage new users – a study in San Francisco, USA, over the period 1986–1992, found that the mean age of clients rose from 36 to 42 years, and that new initiates fell from 3 per cent to 1 per cent (Watters *et al.* 1994). In another study from the USA no increase in discarded syringes was found after the opening of a needle exchange programme (Doherty *et al.* 1997) or at two-year follow-up (Doherty *et al.* 2000).

Impact of needle exchange

Britain would seem to have avoided a rapid rise in HIV rates, as has been seen in other countries. HIV rates remain low among injecting drug users in the UK, compared with other European countries and, as Stimson concludes, 'drug users can change their health behaviour, given both the opportunity, equipment, knowledge and encouragement' (Stimson 1995).

Internationally, needle exchange has been shown to have an impact on many levels. A lowering in the rate of sharing has been noted by a number of researchers (Hartgers *et al.* 1989; Heimer *et al.* 1998; Cox *et al.* 2000) and reduction in injecting drug users' risk of HIV infection (Donoghoe *et al.* 1989; Stimson *et al.* 1988a). In a study of 52 cities without needle exchange schemes and 29 with them, HIV infection rates decreased in cities with schemes and increased in cities without (Hurley *et al.* 1997). Recent government statistics indicate that sharing is still a concern with significant proportions of injectors reporting recently sharing injecting paraphernalia (Department of Health 2001).

In terms of sexual risk, the degree of behaviour change has not matched that seen with change in injecting risk behaviour (Stimson 1992). In the study of the needle exchange pilot in 1987/88, Stimson noted that it was difficult to discuss sexual behaviour with clients at needle exchanges (Stimson *et al.* 1988). Little change in sexual behaviour was noted in one year, in a study of needle exchange clients in central London, although their condom use was quite high and associated with the number of sexual partners (Hart *et al.* 1989). However, needle exchange attenders have been shown to have a greater use of condoms than non-attenders, with casual sexual partners (Frischer and Elliott 1993) and in a study of Welsh needle exchanges, 44 per cent of attenders compared to 61 per cent of non-attenders reported 'some use of condoms' (Keene *et al.* 1993).

The future

While the provision of clean injecting equipment in exchange for used equipment can be seen as the cornerstone of needle exchange, and needle exchange at the very heart of harm minimisation, it is also important to recognise it as part of a paradigm shift that occurred during the 1980s and 1990s – a shift from a focus on drug treatment and abstinence towards a focus on preventing infection. Many of the treatments and services provided by needle exchanges have reached further than providing clean injecting paraphernalia and advice on safer injecting and safer sex. They have allowed there to be a focus on other issues which affect drug users such as their general health and social and legal welfare.

Because a decentralised approach has allowed services to develop to meet local needs, there is a diversity of approaches to how services are run, where they are located both geographically and institutionally and the variety of services they provide in the UK. Little is known about the aims, range and availability of services offered in particular by non-pharmacy-based schemes, and the methods used by needle exchange workers to encourage safer injecting and sexual practices. The most comprehensive data on needle and syringe distribution comes from a 1997 survey (Parsons *et al.*, 2002), in which it was estimated that 27 million syringes were distributed annually in the UK. National data from all needle exchange outlets are not available regarding the demographics of attenders, the type and amount of equipment distributed and how it is disposed of. And this combined with a lack of evidence relating to the effectiveness of many of the interventions provided may leave needle exchange in a weak position. This is especially significant with regard to hepatitis C. Despite the existence of needle exchanges, there exists a relatively high prevalence of the disease among injectors, many of whom use needle exchanges. The danger is that those opponents of needle exchange may seek to use data such as that on hepatitis C rates to promote the closure of needle exchanges. However, what is necessary is a clearer understanding of the relationship between hepatitis C and injecting paraphernalia, which will inform an evidence-based approach, and an expansion in the harm reduction messages provided by exchanges to include information about the dangers of sharing injecting equipment, including paraphernalia such as filters, swabs, water and spoons, and to ensure injecting takes place in a clean environment. A recent change to UK law has made it legal to supply certain additional paraphernalia.

One of the consequences of a 'British' decentralised approach to needle exchange is that there is now an immense amount of variation in service provision. It is probably timely for a national review of needle exchange which would seek to uncover examples of excellent practice and innovative interventions, suitable for commendation and dissemination, as well as the evaluation of the more routine activities.

References

Berridge, V. and Strong, P. (1991). AIDS in the UK: contemporary history and the study of policy. *Twentieth Century British History*, 2, 150–174.

Council of the RPSGB (1993). Guidelines for pharmacists involved in schemes to supply clean needles and syringes. *Pharmaceutical Journal*, 251, 20.

Cox, G. M., Lawless, M. C., Cassin, S. P. and Geoghegan, T. W. (2000). Syringe exchanges: a public health response to problem drug use. *Irish Medical Journal*, 93, 143–146.

Day, P. and Klein, R. (1990). Interpreting the unexpected: the case of AIDS policy making in Britain. *Journal of Public Policy*, 9, 337–353.

Department of Health (2001). Statistics from the regional drug misuse databases on drug misusers in treatment in England, 2000/01. Statistical Bulletin 2001/33. Department of Health, London.

Doherty, M. C., Garfein, R. S., Vlahov, D., Junge, B., Rathouz, P. J., Galai, N., Anthony, J. C. and Beilenson, P. (1997). Discarded needles do not increase soon after the opening of a needle exchange program. *American Journal of Epidemiology*, 145, 730–737.

Doherty, M. C., Junge, B., Rathouz, P., Garfein, R. S., Riley, E. and Vlahov, D. (2000). The effect of a needle exchange program on numbers of discarded needles: a 2-year follow-up. *American Journal of Public Health*, 90, 936–939.

Dolan, K., Stimson, G. V. and Donoghoe, M. C. (1993). Reductions in HIV risk behaviour and stable HIV prevalence in syringe-exchange clients and other injectors in England. *Drug and Alcohol Review*, 12, 133–142.

Donoghoe, M. C., Stimson, G. V. and Dolan, K. A. (1989). Sexual behaviour of injecting drug users and associated risks of HIV infection for non-injecting sexual partners. *AIDS Care*, 1, 51–58.

Donoghoe, M. C., Stimson, G. V. and Dolan, K. (1992). *Syringe exchange in England: an overview*. Tufnell Press, London.

Frischer, M. and Elliott, L. (1993). Discriminating needle exchange attenders from non-attenders. *Addiction*, 88, 681–687.

Guydish, J., Bucardo, J., Young, M., Woods, W., Grinstead, O. and Clark, W. (1993). Evaluating needle exchange: are there negative effects? *AIDS*, 7, 871–876.

Hart, G. J., Carvell, A. L., Woodward, N., Johnson, A. M., Williams, P. and Parry, J. V. (1989). Evaluation of needle exchange in central London: behaviour change and anti-HIV status over one year. *AIDS*, 3, 261–265.

Hartgers, C., Buning, E. C., van Santen, G. W., Verster, A. D. and Coutinho, R. A. (1989). The impact of the needle and syringe exchange programme in Amsterdam in injecting risk behaviour, *AIDS*, 3, 571–576.

Heimer, R., Khoshnood, K., Bigg, D., Guydish, J. and Junge, B. (1998). Syringe use and reuse: effects of syringe exchange programs in four cities. *Journal of Acquired Immunodeficiency Syndromes and Human Retrovirology*, 18 (Suppl. 1): S37–S44.

Hurley, S. F., Jolley, D. J. and Kaldor, J. M. (1997). Effectiveness of needle-exchange programmes for prevention of HIV infection. *Lancet*, 349, 1797–1800.

Keene, J., Stimson, G. V., Jones, S. and Parry-Langdon, N. (1993). Evaluation of syringe exchange for HIV prevention among injecting drug users in rural and urban areas of Wales. *Addiction*, 88, 1063–1070.

Lart, R. and Stimson, G. V. (1990). National survey of syringe exchange schemes in England. *British Journal of Addiction*, 85, 1433–1443.

Macht, D. I. (1916). The history of intravenous and subcutaneous injecting of drugs. *Journal of the American Medical Association*, LXVI.

McKeganey, N. and Barnard, M. (1992). *AIDS, drugs and sexual risk: lives in the balance*, Open University Press, Buckingham, England.

Parsons, J., Hickman, M., Turnbull, P. J., McSweeney, T., Stimson, G. V., Judd, A. and Roberts, K. (2002). Over a decade of syringe exchange: results from 1997 UK survey. *Addiction*, 97, 845–850.

Parsons, J., Sheridan, J., Turnbull, P., Lovell, S., Avendano, M., Stimson, G. and Strang, J. (1999). *The implementation, development and delivery of pharmacy-based needle exchange schemes in north and south Thames*. The Centre for Research on Drugs and Health Behaviour, London.

Rezza, G., Rota, M. C., Buning, E., Hausser, D., O'Hare, P. and Power, R. (1994). Assessing HIV prevention among injecting drug users in European Community countries: a review. *Soz Paventivmed*, 37 (suppl.) S61–S78.

Robertson, J. R., Bucknall, A. B., Welsby, P. D., Roberts, J. J., Inglis, J. M., Peutherer, J. F. and Brettle, R. P. (1986). Epidemic of AIDS-related virus (HTLV-III/LAV) infection among intravenous drug abusers. *British Medical Journal*, 292, 527–529.

RPSGB (Council of) (1982). Sale of syringes. *Pharmaceutical Journal*, 228, 692.

RPSGB (Council of) (1986). Council statement: sale of hypodermic syringes and needles. *Pharmaceutical Journal*, 236, 205.

Sheridan, J., Lovell, S., Turnbull, P., Parsons, J., Stimson, G. and Strang, J. (2000). Pharmacy-based needle exchange (PBNX) schemes in south east England: a survey of service providers. *Addiction*, 95, 1551–1560.

Sheridan, J., Strang, J., Barber, N. and Glanz, A. (1996). Role of community pharmacies in relation to HIV prevention and drug misuse: findings from the 1995 national survey in England and Wales. *British Medical Journal*, 313, 272–274.

Stimson, G. V. (1992). Drug injecting and HIV infection: new directions for social science research. *International Journal of the Addictions*, 27, 142–163.

Stimson, G. V. (1995). AIDS and injecting drug use in the United Kingdom, 1987–1993: the policy response and the prevention of the epidemic. *Social Science and Medicine*, 41, 699–716.

Stimson, G. V., Alldritt, L., Dolan, K. and Donoghoe, M. (1988). Syringe exchange schemes for drug users in England and Scotland. *British Medical Journal*, 296, 1717–1719.

Watters, J. K., Estilo, M. J., Clark, G. L. and Lorvick, J. (1994). Syringe and needle exchange as HIV/AIDS prevention for injection drug users. *Journal of the American Medical Association*, 271, 115–120.

Wolk, J., Wodak, A., Guinan, J. J., Macaskill, P. and Simpson, J. M. (1990). The effect of a needle and syringe exchange on a methadone maintenance unit. *British Journal of Addiction*, 85, 1445–1450.

Chapter 13

The emergence of city-wide public health responses to the drugs problem

Laurence Gruer

'Public health' has been defined as 'the science and art of preventing disease, prolonging life and promoting health through the organised efforts of society' (Secretary of State, 1988). This chapter will examine how just such a combination of science, art and organising can be used successfully to tackle drug misuse at the city level. Glasgow will be taken as the main illustration but the important influence of other cities will be highlighted.

Over the past 25 years, cities across the globe have experienced an unprecedented explosion of drug misuse. The United Kingdom is no exception. Whilst the reasons for the surge in drug misuse are complex, it is easy to understand why it thrives in cities. They are home to many beset by poverty, despair or boredom for whom drugs offer solace, escape or excitement. Drugs can be efficiently delivered, sold and distributed and illicit activity pass unnoticed. Money for buying drugs can be efficiently generated by shoplifting, car theft, prostitution and fraud and laundered through businesses and banks.

Just as the city is fertile ground for drug misuse, so, in principle, can it offer the potential for an organised response. Information gathering, planning and organising all tend to be more readily achieved in cities than in sparsely populated rural areas. However, the opportunities for a city-wide response will depend upon the wider political, legislative and cultural environment. In tackling its drug problems, a city has to conform to government policy and national laws. These may differ markedly from country to country. It also needs to work within existing institutions such as local government and health services. Thus, what is readily possible in one country may be difficult or impossible in another. Nevertheless, tackling drug misuse at the city level presents common challenges and opportunities wherever it might be. Four ingredients are essential and will be examined in turn:

1   A city-wide strategy
2   Political consent and support
3   Adequate resources
4   Effective city-wide and centralised services

The roots of the problem

Glasgow has a current population of around 620,000. Over the past 30 years, its traditional heavy industries have all but vanished, leading to mass unemployment. Its infamous slums of the nineteenth and early twentieth centuries were replaced in the 1950s and 1960s by high-rise flats and vast peripheral council housing estates. It is here that drug misuse has become a way of life for many, supported by flourishing networks of drug dealers and a thriving black economy based on stolen goods.

The modern wave of drug misuse in Glasgow began in 1981. During that year, the number of new heroin addicts seen at the city's two main drug clinics soared from 34 to 174 (Ditton and Speirits, 1982). With too few staff, and no supporting services, they were quickly overwhelmed. They abandoned methadone prescribing and became a 'drug-free' enclave. Over the next five years the number of heroin injectors continued to escalate. Whereas previously addicts were from a variety of backgrounds (Bennie and Sclare, 1966), most were now young and unemployed from the most deprived parts of the city. Without specialist help, social work departments, general practitioners and accident and emergency departments struggled to respond. The number of cases of hepatitis B among young drug injectors rose, heralding worse to come (Gruer et al., 1991).

Late in 1985 the news broke that 38 per cent of a sample of drug injectors in nearby Edinburgh were infected with HIV (Peutherer et al., 1985). The nightmare had crossed the Atlantic (Robertson et al., 1986). Fearing heterosexual transmission from drug injectors to the wider community, the nation panicked. Within weeks, a government advisory group had been set up. Drawing their inspiration from the experience in Amsterdam (Buning et al., 1986), the group's report recommended the establishment of pilot needle exchanges in Edinburgh, Glasgow and Dundee (Scottish Home and Health Department, 1986). Exchanges were also being set up in a number of English cities including Liverpool, London, Sheffield and Bradford.

In 1987, another government working group considered how the National Health Service in Scotland could cope with people with HIV and AIDS (Scottish Home and Health Department, 1987). Three regional HIV care centres were set up. Meanwhile, the Royal Pharmaceutical Society relaxed its restrictions on the sale of injecting equipment by community pharmacists, providing injectors in some areas with easier access to clean needles and syringes. A clarion call for action to prevent the spread of HIV among drug injectors came from the Advisory Council on the Misuse of Drugs (1988).

Creating a city-wide strategy

Whilst these were important responses, they did not represent a comprehensive approach either to HIV infection or to drug misuse. Nevertheless, the government were surprisingly reluctant to examine the wider strategic implications of HIV on drug misuse in Scotland. Faced with what he saw as a dangerous policy vacuum, Fred Edwards, the Director of Social Work for Strathclyde Regional Council, whose department covered Glasgow and much of the west of Scotland, acted. He persuaded the four constituent health authorities in Strathclyde, including Greater Glasgow, to join him in a multi-agency working group to draw up a comprehensive strategy for tackling HIV and drug injecting. Although relevant to the whole of the region, the strategy's main focus was on Glasgow where most drug misusers lived. Their report provided a clear line of attack for the next five years (Strathclyde Regional Council, 1988). Key recommendations included the need for:

1   sources of sterile needles and syringes for drug injectors;
2   services for street prostitutes providing free condoms and drugs advice and services;
3   community-based and residential drug projects; and
4   substitute prescribing for heroin injectors when indicated.

Political consent and support

A key achievement of this report was to win the support of all the main agencies including the health authorities, the local authorities responsible for social work, education, environmental health, the police and the voluntary sector. This provided the essential local political backing for taking action. It was also explicitly recognised that unless agencies worked in partnership, there would be chaos and discord. Four years later, a Scottish strategy for HIV prevention was finally published (Scottish Office, 1992). A Scottish drug misuse strategy was published in 1994 (Scottish Office, 1994), followed by a similar report for England (HM Government, 1995) leading to the establishment of Drug Action Teams (DAT) in every health authority area, each charged with producing a local drug misuse strategy. The Greater Glasgow DAT's first strategy came out in 1995 and a second in 1999. With the exception of a short period of disunity following local government reorganisation in 1996, a high level of political consensus on tackling both the drug problem and HIV in Glasgow has been sustained since 1988. This has provided the foundation for successful joint work between the health service and local government services, notably social work.

Adequate resources

Without the means to do so, implementing a strategy, however good it looks on paper, will be difficult or impossible. Fortunately, from 1985 onwards, Central Government did begin to make funds available. First there were grants to establish small community drug projects, then small amounts for needle exchange and larger sums for HIV treatment services. In addition, Strathclyde Regional Council, spurred on by their charismatic Director of Social Work, invested new money in social care services for drug misusers. By the early 1990s, substantial ring-fenced funds were being made available. These have proved crucial in enabling a wide range of initiatives to get off the ground. By 1998, Greater Glasgow Health Board and Glasgow City Council were between them spending around £10 million annually on drug misuse services.

Implementing effective city-wide and centralised services

Even with a strategy, political commitment and additional resources, the problems are far from over. It is in attempting to develop and implement services capable of making a real impact that the true challenges lie. In developing the public health response to drug misuse in Greater Glasgow since 1987, three clear objectives were established:

1   to reduce the extent of sharing used injecting equipment;
2   to reduce the prevalence and frequency of injecting; and
3   to reduce the extent of drug misuse.

To measure how far such objectives are being achieved needs good information. Some data on the prevalence of HIV among drug injectors in Glasgow were available from 1987 but it was not until 1990 that more representative samples of drug injectors could be tested for HIV. These confirmed that the prevalence of HIV peaked at around 5 per cent in 1987 but has remained at around 1 per cent since 1989 (Frischer et al., 1992). Estimating the prevalence of drug injecting was more difficult. However, creative use of the capture–recapture method of estimating wild animal populations suggested there were around 8,500 drug injectors in Greater Glasgow in 1990 (Frischer et al., 1991). Around 70 per cent were male and most were in their twenties. Further research revealed the types of drugs used: a wide range of opiates, benzodiazepines and stimulants (Rhodes et al., 1993). Good information has allowed planning and service implementation to be based on reasonably solid evidence and has helped maintain the support of senior managers, health authority board members and local authority councillors.

Needle exchange

Developing successful city-wide services requires a combination of inspiration, persistence and luck. Take needle exchange, for example. The first pilot needle exchange in Glasgow was set up in the gatehouse of a hospital that was relatively inaccessible to almost everyone. It was only open on two afternoons a week for two and a half hours each afternoon, when most injectors would be busy dealing or scoring. For the first six months it was picketed by angry locals and used by a handful of addicts. It was a failure. The breakthrough came in January 1989 when an evening needle exchange was quietly opened in a drug project in the notorious Easterhouse housing estate. It was a local, accessible service advertised by word of mouth. Its success was immediate and the premises quickly proved too small. Five months later, the exchange was transferred to the nearby health centre which could be used in the evening without interfering with daytime services. It was soon attended by around 100 clients each evening. We now had a service model that could be replicated in other parts of the city where drug injecting was most prevalent. In preparing for each new exchange, there was extensive public consultation to avoid the demonstrations that marred the early days. A crucial factor in achieving local community support was the remarkably high proportions of used needles and syringes that were returned. This helped allay the fears of local residents that needle exchanges would lead to large numbers of needles and syringes being discarded in public places. In all, seven community-based exchanges were established (Gruer et al., 1993). In one area, the home of Glasgow Rangers, the needle exchange proposal became a political football between Labour and the Scottish National Party candidates and was 'booted out of the park'. To ensure uniform standards and staffing, the exchange service was co-ordinated centrally. A system of continuous audit enabled the performance of each exchange to be carefully monitored. Evidence was obtained that needle exchange attenders were less likely to borrow used equipment than non-attenders and overall sharing rates had diminished (Frischer et al., 1993b).

Efforts to establish a city-wide network of needle exchanges in community pharmacies were, however, thwarted. After having seen successful schemes in Bradford and Sheffield, plans were drawn up and approved by Greater Glasgow Health Board in 1989. A survey showed that substantial numbers of pharmacists who did not wish to sell needles and syringes were prepared to operate an exchange. However, the scheme was rejected by the Scottish Health Minister who ruled that the provision of needles and syringes through community pharmacies should be by 'a normal commercial transaction'. By the time the government changed its mind in 1992, community pharmacists' attitudes had hardened and relatively few joined the scheme. An opportunity had been lost.

Methadone

Whilst there was good evidence of reducing levels of equipment sharing, we were making no impact on the extent of drug injecting. As a result, other injecting-related problems were common, including abscesses, venous and arterial thrombosis, gangrene and infective endocarditis (Scott et al., 1992).

Overdose among drug injectors had become the most frequent cause of death in Glasgow among 15–35-year-olds (Frischer *et al.*, 1993a).

Despite the evidence that methadone maintenance was the most reliable way of reducing heroin injecting, by 1992 virtually the only drug injectors in Glasgow to receive methadone had HIV infection and were managed by infectious disease physicians! The city's addiction psychiatrists steadfastly refused to use methadone, citing the bitter experience of the early 1980s. Other than offering detoxification – usually unsuccessful – they gave general practitioners little meaningful assistance. Left to fend for themselves, GPs oscillated from complete rejection and exclusion of addicts from their lists to dangerous complicity with patients demanding prescriptions for buprenorphine, dihydrocodeine or temazepam. Prescribed drugs were widely abused. The parents of drug injectors organised themselves into vociferous family support groups, expressing their outrage at the perceived naivety and incompetence of general practitioners.

For a way out of this mess, inspiration was found in nearby Edinburgh and within our midst. Faced with a major HIV epidemic among drug injectors, Dr Judy Greenwood had established a specialist community drug problem service in Edinburgh which took referrals from general practitioners and operated a system of shared care (Greenwood, 1990). The service would assess the patient and initiate treatment with methadone where appropriate. Once stabilised, the patient would be returned to the care of his or her GP. The CDPS (Community Drug Problem Service) had achieved remarkable success in encouraging a high proportion of GPs in Edinburgh to treat patients with methadone, leading to a large reduction in the proportion of opiate addicts in Edinburgh who were injecting (Greenwood, 1996). Plans for a similar service in Glasgow were drawn up in 1992. At around the same time, several GPs in Glasgow began using methadone in a more systematic way. They used patient contracts, saw drug-misusing patients at a separate clinic and closely involved drug workers in their ongoing care. Another important innovation – to ensure compliance and avoid diversion – was to arrange for patients to consume their methadone under the supervision of the dispensing pharmacist. Early results were extremely encouraging (Wilson *et al.*, 1994). Nevertheless, it was clear that doing this type of work took up a lot of time. This, GPs argued, merited additional payment. A working group involving the health board and the Local Medical Committee for GPs therefore drew up proposals for a GP Drug Misuse Clinic Scheme. Under the scheme, GPs would agree to follow clinical guidelines, work in partnership with drug workers or counsellors, attend training seminars and submit data. In return, they would be paid extra. It was agreed that methadone should always be taken under supervision until the GP was confident it would not be misused, and that prescribing temazepam or dihydrocodeine to drug misusers in the scheme should be prohibited.

The Glasgow Drug Problem Service (GDPS) and the GP Drug Misuse Clinic Scheme were launched early in 1994 and both were an instant success

(Burnett *et al.*, 1994; Gruer *et al.*, 1997). Within six months of starting, the GDPS had received over 1,000 referrals and had to close its doors for six months to deal with the backlog. Since then it has handled 1,200–1,500 referrals a year from more than 70 per cent of all GPs in the Greater Glasgow area. By transforming many of their most problematic patients, Dr Bob Scott, the director of the GDPS, was able to win the hearts and minds of many GPs who previously had been steadfastly against the use of methadone.

Thirty-nine GPs signed up at the start of the Drug Misuse Clinic Scheme. By 1999, there were more than 130, representing over one-third of all practices. During the first five years no GP decided to leave the scheme except for retirement or ill-health. The number of patients treated in the scheme rose from 1,200 in 1994/95 to 3,580 in 1998/99. The commitment of community pharmacists and drug workers to the scheme was even more impressive. A survey undertaken in early 1994 found that 97 (46 per cent) of the city's community pharmacies were dispensing methadone and 43 (20 per cent) were voluntarily supervising the daily consumption of methadone. Since then, the number of pharmacies dispensing methadone has increased to 189 (89 per cent), and 145 (68 per cent) have contracted with the Health Board to supervise its consumption (Roberts *et al.*, 1998). All 13 community-based drug projects in Greater Glasgow are now committed to providing counselling and support for clients receiving methadone. In many cases, joint clinics between the general practitioner and the drug worker are held, either in the GP's surgery or on the drug project's premises. Cohort and cross-sectional studies have demonstrated that most patients treated with methadone in the city under these arrangements show great improvements in health and social functioning compared with their pre-treatment state (Gruer *et al.*, 1998). There is also evidence that, compared with Edinburgh where supervised methadone was not introduced until late 1997, both the incidence of methadone-related deaths and the proportion of addicts using street methadone have been much lower in Glasgow (Information and Statistics Division, 1999). The methadone programme in Glasgow has also had a dramatic effect on property crime (Barr *et al.*, 1997).

Centralised specialist services

Another type of city-wide response is the centralised specialist service – five are briefly described.

The Department of Infection

Drug injecting results in a high risk of many types of infection. It is thus essential to have a specialist team capable of providing both immediate care for acute life-threatening infections and longer-term management of chronic infections, notably HIV and hepatitis C. Such services have a key role to play, not only in providing individual patient care but also in protecting the wider public health. A high proportion of cases of drug injecting-related HIV in Glasgow have been diagnosed and subsequently followed up by the Department of Infection where many have been treated with long-term methadone maintenance. Many have reduced or stopped injecting, thereby cutting the risk of transmission of HIV to other drug injectors. This has probably been a key factor in maintaining a low prevalence of HIV among drug injectors in Glasgow.

Obstetric and gynaecological services

Pregnancy in a drug injector is rarely straightforward. Dealing with chaotic drug use and the myriad associated social problems is a task well beyond the inclination and capability of a normal obstetric unit. In the absence of effective specialist care, a distraught mother and a sick baby taken into care are the likely outcomes. Since 1990 the Glasgow Women's Reproductive Health Service has provided a comprehensive obstetric and gynaecological service for women with social problems of which drug misuse is the most common. Staffed by doctors and midwives, it functions through five community-based clinics in areas of high drug misuse prevalence, with an eight-bedded unit in a city centre maternity hospital. Drug detoxification or maintenance regimes are offered where appropriate and there is close liaison with social work and other services for women. The outcome of pregnancy for drug-misusing women managed by the service has been superior to that reported in areas without such a service (Hepburn, 1993).

Drop-in centre for female street prostitutes

Since 1989, Greater Glasgow Health Board and the Social Work Department have jointly operated a service for female street prostitutes in the city centre. Staffed by social workers, nurses and doctors, it opens six nights a week for free condoms, needles and syringes, first aid and other basic health care and advice on health and social problems. A hepatitis B immunisation pro-gramme, cervical screening and contraceptive services are also provided. Over 90 per cent of the 35–50 attenders per evening are female drug injectors, many of whom have severe physical and mental health problems but whose ability to access adequate health and social care elsewhere is often extremely limited (Carr et al., 1996).

Glasgow drug crisis centre

The impetus for a crisis centre came initially from parents of drug addicts, critical of the lack of help from existing services when they were most needed. Planning for the centre by a joint social work/health board group began in

1989. It was agreed that the service should be available to all comers, twenty-four hours a day. A visit to the City Roads drug crisis project in London was helpful but we felt that an open-door facility was essential and nothing similar then existed in the UK. As there was strong local political agreement that a crisis centre was needed, obtaining funding was relatively straightforward. Much more difficult was finding an appropriate site. This had to be near the city centre, with good transport links and enough space for a twelve-bedded unit, walk-in consulting and counselling rooms, leisure facilities and office space. A number of potential sites had to be discounted due to the opposition of local residents. Finally, an old school was selected as the best option. A second challenge was to ensure that the centre would be properly managed and staffed. When no suitable local candidates could be found, a contract to manage the project was agreed with Turning Point, one of the UK's largest and most experienced organisations in this field.

Since it opened in 1994, the centre has fully justified its existence. In its first four years, the twelve beds (maximum three weeks' stay) have always run at over 90 per cent occupancy. In 1997/98, the open access, 'one-stop' facility was used by well over 3,000 individuals. Homelessness, physical and mental ill-health, and legal and child-care issues are the most common problems, often in combination. A major part of the centre's work is to find ways of establishing ongoing treatment and support through local community drug services, general practitioners and residential services. A need for an in-house needle exchange service was identified during the first two years. Open from 1997, it quickly became the busiest needle exchange in Britain by virtue of its city centre location and 24-hour availability. The centre initially lacked good liaison with mental health services but this has now been rectified.

Residential and community-based rehabilitation services

An important element of any comprehensive response to drug misuse and dependence is the provision of support for people aiming to achieve and sustain abstinence. A variety of service models are available in Glasgow including the Minnesota Model and Narcotics Anonymous, the Phoenix House Therapeutic Community and locally developed approaches centred on sport and fitness. Whilst there are successes, relapse rates are extremely high. Rarely is it possible for individuals to escape completely from a social and cultural environment pervaded by drug taking. The opportunities for recovering drug users to find legitimate paid work are currently extremely limited.

A gloomy outlook

Yes, an HIV epidemic has been averted, many drug-related deaths avoided and hundreds of thousands of crimes prevented. If it were not for the action and services outlined here, the situation would have been much worse. But while much has been done to alleviate individual suffering and protect the public health, the root causes remain. With the worst drug problems in Glasgow strongly related to socio-economic deprivation (Advisory Council on the Misuse of Drugs, 1998), it is unlikely that much overall improvement will be possible without substantial regeneration of deprived areas and the creation of worthwhile employment opportunities for the young people who live there. Despite the present government's undoubted commitment to reducing social exclusion and alleviating poverty, the long-term outlook for many parts of Glasgow and similar cities is not hopeful. To a large extent the initiatives described here, however successful in their own terms, are simply papering over the cracks. Major renovation is required.

References

Advisory Council on the Misuse of Drugs (1988). AIDS and Drug Misuse Part 1 (London, HMSO).

Advisory Council on the Misuse of Drugs (1998). Drug Misuse and the Environment (London, Home Office).

Barr, C., Farquhar, D., Taylor, A., Gruer, L. and Frischer, M. (1997). The impact of methadone on crime in Glasgow, *Euromethwork Newsletter*, 11, 13–14.

Bennie, E. and Sclare, A. (1966). Heroin addiction in Glasgow, *Scottish Medical Journal*, 11, 319–21.

Buning, E., Coutinho, R., Van Brussel, G., Van Sarten, G. *et al.* (1986). Preventing AIDS in drug addicts in Amsterdam, *Lancet*, i, 1435.

Burnett, S., Scott, R., Cameron, J., Elliott, L. and Gruer, L. (1994). The Glasgow Drug Problem Service, *Scottish Medicine*, 14, 12–13.

Carr, S., Goldberg, D., Elliott, L., Green, S., Mackie, C. and Gruer, L. (1996). A primary health care service for Glasgow street sex workers – 6 years experience of the Drop-in Centre 1989–1994, *AIDS Care*, 8, 489–97.

Ditton, J. and Speirits, K. (1982). The new wave of heroin addiction in Britain, *Sociology*, 16, 595–98.

Frischer, M., Bloor, M., Finlay, A. *et al.* (1991). A new method of estimating prevalence of injecting drug use in an urban population: results from a Scottish city, *International Journal of Epidemiology*, 20, 997–1000.

Frischer, M., Green, S., Goldberg, D., Haw, S. *et al.* (1992). Estimates of HIV infection among injecting drug users in Glasgow 1985–1990, *AIDS*, 6, 1371–75.

Frischer, M., Bloor, M., Goldberg, D., Dark, J., Green, S. and McKeganey, N. (1993a). Mortality among injecting drug users: a critical re-appraisal, *Epidemiology and Community Health*, 47, 59–63.

Frischer, M., Elliott, L., Taylor, A., Goldberg, D., Green, S., Gruer, L., Cameron, J., McKeganey, N. and Bloor, M. (1993b). Do needle exchanges help to control the spread of HIV among injecting drug users? *AIDS*, 7, 1677–90.

Greenwood, J. (1990). Creating a new drug service in Edinburgh, *British Medical Journal*, 300, 587–89.

Greenwood, J. (1996). Six years of sharing the care of Edinburgh drug users, *Psychiatric Bulletin*, 20, 8–11.

Gruer, L., Peedie, M., Carrington, D., Clements, G. and Follett, E. (1991). Distribution of HIV and acute hepatitis B infection among drug injectors in Glasgow, *International Journal of STD and AIDS*, 2, 356–58.

Gruer, L., Cameron, J. and Elliott, L. (1993). Building a city-wide service for exchanging needles and syringes, *British Medical Journal*, 306, 1394–97.

Gruer, L., Wilson, P., Scott, R., Elliott, L. *et al.* (1997). General practitioner centred scheme for treatment of opiate dependent drug injectors in Glasgow, *British Medical Journal*, 314, 1730–35.

Gruer, L., Taylor, A., Elliott, L., Scott, R., Frischer, M. and Goldberg, D. (1998). The Impact of Methadone in Glasgow Study. Final report (Edinburgh, Chief Scientist Office).

Hepburn, M. (1993). Drug misuse in pregnancy, *British Journal of Hospital Medicine*, 49, 51–55.

HM Government (1995). Tackling Drugs Together: A Strategy for England 1995–1998 (London, HMSO).

Information and Statistics Division (1999). Drug Misuse Statistics Scotland, 1998 Bulletin (Edinburgh).

Peutherer, J., Edmond, E., Simmonds, P., Dickson, J. and Bath, G. (1985). HTLV-III antibody in Edinburgh drug addicts. *Lancet*, ii, 1129.

Rhodes, T., Bloor, M., Donoghoe, M. *et al.* (1993). HIV prevalence and HIV risk behaviour among injecting drug users in London and Glasgow, *AIDS Care*, 5, 413–25.

Roberts, K., McNulty, H., Gruer, L., Scott, R. and Bryson, S. (1998). The role of Glasgow pharmacists in the management of drug misuse, *International Journal of Drug Policy*, 9, 187–94.

Robertson, J. R., Bucknall, A. B. V., Welsby, P. D., Roberts, J. J. K., Inglis, J. M., Pentherer, J. F. *et al.* (1986). Epidemic of AIDS related virus infection among intravenous drug abusers, *British Medical Journal*, 292, 527–29.

Scott, R., Woodburn, K. R., Reid, D. B., Maraj, B., Going, J., Gilmour, D. G. *et al.* (1992). Intra-arterial temazepam, *British Medical Journal*, 304, 1630.

Scottish Home and Health Department (1986). HIV Infection in Scotland: Report of the Scottish Committee on HIV Infection and Intravenous Drug Misuse, The McClelland Report (Edinburgh).

Scottish Home and Health Department (1987). Report of the National Working Party on Health Service Implications of HIV Infection, The Tayler Report (Edinburgh).

Scottish Office (1992). HIV and AIDS in Scotland: Prevention the Key (Edinburgh, HMSO).

Scottish Office (1994). Drug Misuse in Scotland: Meeting the Challenge: Report of a Ministerial Drugs Task Force (Edinburgh, HMSO).

Secretary of State (1988). Public Health in England: the report of the Committee of Inquiry into the future developments of the public health function, The Acheson Report (London, HMSO).

Strathclyde Regional Council (1988). HIV Infection and AIDS: Towards an Inter-agency Strategy in Strathclyde (Glasgow).

Wilson, P., Watson, R. and Ralston, G. E. (1994). Methadone maintenance in general practice: patients, workload and outcomes, *British Medical Journal*, 309, 691–94.

Chapter 14

Narcotics Anonymous (NA) in Britain

The stepping up of the phenomenon

Brian Wells

(This chapter draws subtantially on the chapter previously written by the author and published in J. Strang and M. Gossop (eds) *Heroin Addiction and Drug Policy: The British System*, Oxford University Press, 1994.)

History

The 12-step fellowships originated in May 1935 when Bill Wilson and Dr Robert Smith, both chronic alcoholics, met in Akron, Ohio, and founded Alcoholics Anonymous (AA). The first 100 members collectively wrote the 'Big Book', the 12 steps and the traditions of AA. AA has always insisted that it exists to provide a recovery programme for those suffering from the illness of 'alcoholism'. Those suffering from other disorders have been encouraged to go elsewhere, leading to a plethora of self-help organisations based upon the 12 steps, including Gamblers Anonymous, Emotions Anonymous, Over-eaters Anonymous, and Paranoids Anonymous (the latter being somewhat difficult to find!).

Narcotics Anonymous (NA) began in California in July 1953, when a group of motorcycle-riding, middle-aged heroin addicts were ejected from their local AA meeting with some acrimony. They altered the first step from 'We admitted that we were powerless over alcohol . . .', to 'We admitted that we were powerless over our addiction . . .', but otherwise retained the steps, the traditions and the entire programme of recovery, applying them to the 'illness of addiction', thus offering the same to persons suffering problems relating to the whole spectrum of mind-altering chemicals.

In the UK, NA was born in 1979 when an ex-drug-using AA member started the first meeting at St George's Hostel, Worlds End, Chelsea. This weekly meeting continued for a year with a gradually increasing attendance. Then a second meeting was started, then a third. Three 'delegates' flew to Memphis and attended an NA Literature Writing and Service Convention. Upon their return in 1981, NA meetings began springing up all over London and in scattered parts of the country, notably Bristol and Weston-super-Mare.

Growth was sporadic and appeared to depend upon local attitudes to 12-step fellowships and in particular the presence of 12-step-based treatment centres, the first of which was Broadway Lodge in Weston-super-Mare.

By 1984 Weston-super-Mare had become an interesting microcosm. There were at least eight NA meetings per week, some of which had mushroomed and just as rapidly folded, largely attended by ex-problem drug users who had left treatment and decided to remain in the area (either resident in a half-way house or living and working locally). At the same time a number of addicts had left treatment prematurely (or been thrown out) who also decided to live locally and continue to use drugs. The town became something of a national centre for drug taking and recovery, to the extent that users would travel from Wales, Bath and Bristol to Weston-super-Mare in order to buy heroin. Many of these 'addicts' had friends who were in the recovery community (perhaps from their treatment peer group) and subsequently 'cleaned up', moving from the using camp to join their companions in recovery.

Elsewhere in the country, attitudes towards the fellowships were more cynical within both 'using' and professional cultures. Thus in Manchester, NA struggled to survive and blamed local professional attitudes as a major cause of the problem. In Liverpool, NA remains minimal, whilst a strong meeting has been flourishing for some 11 years, across the river in Birkenhead. As other treatment centres opened (mainly in southern England) so local NA flourished, whereas in Birmingham and Newcastle attendance has remained poor.

A London office was acquired, the service structure (quite different from that of AA) was developed and NA spread throughout the UK during the mid-1980s, so that by 1991 there were 223 weekly meetings attended by 'recovering addicts' in Britain. By 2004 there were well over 500 NA meetings in the UK, 135 of which were in Greater London. Meetings have also been started in a variety of prisons as well as a number of 'non-twelve-step' treatment centres. Within NA itself there is a tendency towards subcultures and 'cliques'. For example, some members prefer to avoid the Chelsea meetings, feeling more comfortable, say, in the East End. In general, mature members are happy to attend anywhere, at any time. As with AA, there is a 'life force' to the meetings, which changes in atmosphere as years go by, some becoming too big, or possibly the result of a personality clash, members starting a new meeting of differing format nearby.

In the USA, NA grew as a classless structure with a small college attending periphery, whereas in the UK, early NA was largely perpetuated by the energies of young people from socially advantaged backgrounds, many of whom had been through fee-paying treatment programmes. Thus early NA in Britain was viewed as existing for the privileged and hence unattractive to many problem drug users, whilst professionals in the field, many of whom had never considered AA as a useful treatment resource, became concerned over what they saw as a 'resource for the private sector', in 'a self-help group for rich people'. Alarm was expressed over such notions as 'the disease concept' and the need for a 'higher power' whilst workers felt that strategies such as 'tough love' and 'total abstinence' were tantamount to 'brain washing'. Many such opinions persist today amongst British drug working professionals, although the balance in NA itself has now shifted to include many addicts from disadvantaged and 'ethnic' backgrounds.

The ideology

NA subscribes to the view that once recreational drug use has become compulsive, the 'addict' has crossed a thin line into a physical, psychological and spiritual illness that can only get worse with continued drug use. The illness is seen as progressive and eventually fatal unless it is arrested by daily abstinence, allowing a process of recovery to begin. 'Addicts' are seen as not responsible for their illness, but 100 per cent responsible for recovery, via the maintenance of abstinence (from all mood-altering chemicals including alcohol) and active work done on the suggested programme of recovery.

Alcohol

Recovery doesn't stop with just being clean. As we abstain from all drugs (and yes this means alcohol and marijuana too) we come face to face with feelings that we never coped with successfully (NA 1989).

Many 'addicts' have had serious problems with alcohol as well as other forms of polydrug taking. Alcohol is seen as 'just another sedative drug' and is frequently referred to in meetings, to the extent that many 'alcoholics' who have had no apparent difficulty with other drugs, prefer the atmosphere of NA to AA meetings. NA tends to be more youthful, more energetic and lively, whilst some would say less stable and less mature. The main factor is probably the age and life experience of the members involved, so the younger drinker is often more attracted to NA. This is, however, not always the case. NA contains many 'elder statesmen' who have had problems with, say, alcohol and benzodiazepines, and who are able to identify more with NA than their local AA counterpart.

The family

The illness is seen as affecting the entire family. Where there has been 'active addiction' over a number of years, family members (including children) often experience distress, unpredictability, violence and legal consequences.

The self-help groups, Alcoholics Anonymous and Families Anonymous (FA) exist for family members of 'alcoholics' and 'addicts', respectively. They are also 12-step fellowships in which family members are encouraged to work their own programme, placing responsibility for recovery from addiction upon the shoulders of the active alcoholic/addict. They are not organisations for people to attend in order to complain about their using/drinking spouse, but rather they exist to offer the same active programme of recovery to family members whose lives have become dysfunctional.

The programme

The suggested programme of recovery involves attendance at NA meetings. These are numerous in urban areas, to be found in hospitals, prisons and other institutions as well as in the community. Meetings vary in their format (speaker meetings, step meetings, topic meetings, etc.) but generally consist of a main speaker sharing his or her experience of addiction and recovery, possibly in relation to a particular topic (relationships, spirituality, etc.) or on one of the 12 steps. The meeting is then opened up for sharing from the floor. Typically, members introduce themselves as 'I'm Fred/Jane, I'm an addict' and then refer to the topic in question. Sometimes , however, sharing simply involves an account of what has happened that day, good times, difficulties, 'here and now events'. There is frequently much gratitude expressed towards the fellowship, and at times newcomers may be forgiven for thinking that they have walked into a room full of fanatics.

Sharing is, in general, supportive, non-judgemental and includes personal identification with the main speaker and his or her subject. Visitors are often surprised at the degree of humour that abounds in meetings, Many members are articulate and psychologically sophisticated, whilst others are shy and less forthcoming. All are supported by the group.

Members are encouraged to attend frequently in the early days in order to become familiar with the jargon, the other members and the various formats, but in particular in order to 'flood' the new member with a process that is likely to be unfamiliar, strange and sometimes frightening. Many new members feel they have entered into something akin to a religious sect, while sharing about personal issues in public is often an alien experience. Relatively few newcomers (or indeed professionals) are able to embrace this programme with enthusiasm if they visit only a few times.

Members are encouraged to get involved, to acquire a sponsor (someone with whom they can discuss their difficulties and perceptions on a one-to-one basis) and to begin to absorb the fundamental NA message which clearly states, 'We support each other in remaining drug free, just one day at a time.'

Telephone numbers are exchanged, post-meeting rendezvous take place, conventions and fundraising events are held. Dances, parties and 'service events' all exist to offer the newcomer a support system within a true fellowship of recovering people that collectively retains the clear focus of daily abstinence.

The 12 steps of NA

Narcotics Anonymous members have followed the 12 steps originated by Alcoholics Anonymous:

1 We admitted that we are powerless over our addiction, that our lives had become unmanageable.
2 We came to believe that a power greater than ourselves could restore us to sanity.
3 We made a decision to turn our will and our lives over to the care of God as we understood him.
4 We made a searching and fearless moral inventory of ourselves.
5 We admitted to God, to ourselves, and to another human being the exact nature of our wrongs.
6 We were entirely ready to have God remove all these defects of character.
7 We humbly asked Him to remove our shortcomings.
8 We made a list of all persons we had harmed, and became willing to make amends to them all.
9 We made direct amends to such people wherever possible, except when to do so would injure them or others.
10 We continued to take personal inventory, and when we were wrong promptly admitted it.
11 We sought through prayer and meditation to improve our conscious contact with God, as we understood Him, praying only for knowledge of His will for us, and the power to carry it out.
12 Having had a spiritual awakening as a result of these steps, we tried to carry this message to addicts and to practise these principles in all our affairs.

NA chose to retain the steps in their original form as written by the early AA members. Some of these members came from the religious Oxford movement and much early AA literature contains a strong religious overtone. It was felt, however, that the steps had stood the test of time and should not therefore be altered.

Much criticism is levelled at NA for its 'quasi-religious' orientation. Reference to God appears in six of the 12 steps, and prayer and meditation are encouraged. NA, however, is not a religious organisation. There is a spiritual component based upon the personal understanding of a 'Power greater than oneself'. This may be the power of the group, the power of nature, love, collectivity, or some force connected with truth and honesty. Feelings of well-being engendered by the process of collective personal growth are often referred to as 'spiritual'. Whilst some members eventually do become involved with 'organised religion' others experiment with forms of meditation, martial arts, yoga, physical exercise, etc., or completely ignore the spirituality suggested by the programme.

The steps encourage a deep understanding of the need for daily abstinence, as well as insight into self. The making of restitution to self and others and the development of a spiritual direction lead to the spread of the recovery message to the still suffering addict: 'We keep what we have by giving it away.'

Many attend NA and pay no attention to the steps. The organisation is used on a number of levels, from enhancement of social contact to what is sometimes seen as 'obsessive' preoccupation with the process of recovery and growth.

Who attends?

'Very simply an addict is a man or woman whose life is controlled by drugs. There is only one requirement for membership, the honest desire to stop using.'

In practice NA membership comprises a variety of persons who have experienced problems relating to drugs. Many have been dependent upon opioids, alcohol, stimulants and sedatives. Some describe a history of chaotic polydrug misuse, whilst others have become concerned over heavy recreational use of cannabis. Overall, males exceed females two-to-one. The attending population varies with geographical location and local drug-taking practices. Central London meetings are likely to include teenagers as well as elderly people dependent upon prescribed benzodiazepines. The atmosphere is variable and it is suggested that newcomers should 'shop around' looking for meetings to which they are attracted.

Affiliation with NA

Initial impressions suggest that those with social confidence and verbal fluency are more likely to affiliate with NA. Whilst further research is needed, it is often surprising that the 'least likely' candidates sometimes become active and valuable NA members. The converse is also true with those 'tipped as likely to succeed' sometimes quite unable to internalise the basics of the programme.

People find NA through mutual friends, old acquaintances, prisons, counsellors, parents and wives who begin attending family fellowships, or sometimes by just wandering in off the street. Sometimes people are simply 'just not ready' to engage. They often return, however, perhaps two years later having 'tried it out their way' eventually deciding to 'come around'. Anecdotally the most powerful influence seems to be that of peer group persuasion and attraction as found in the fellowship itself and as used more formally in the 12-step-based treatment.

Treatment

The most common form of treatment in the USA is abstinence-based and makes use of AA/NA principles. In the USA there were literally thousands of 28-day residential programmes that encouraged problem drug users/drinkers to understand themselves as people with an illness who need to get well, via abstinence and attendance at 12-step fellowships. In the UK this became known as the Minnesota Model (see Wells 1987; Cook 1988). In the USA many such centres folded in the 1990s as a result of insurance cutbacks and 'managed care'.

Such treatment centres are to be found in the private and charitable sectors, whilst a diluted version is sometimes practised in National Health Service (NHS) alcohol and addiction units. Twelve-step treatment centres may be residential, with programmes lasting from 21 to 56 days. They may be out-patient or day-care with a number of 'half-way houses' available. Some centres offer a family programme in which family members spend a residential period, followed by attendance at family fellowships to deal with their own difficulties. Most centres ask the family to attend at weekends, to be part of the addict's recovery programme both during and after treatment.

An entire book is being written (by an NA member) about the development of the Minnesota Model treatment centres. From Broadway Lodge which opened in 1974, a plethora of centres have developed. The issue of funding has been a constant and sometimes fatal area of difficulty, with some centres having been forced to close within weeks of having opened. Different centres have different styles, with some being purely available to fee-paying patients or those with insurance. Others have registered as nursing homes and take patients on 'assisted place' receiving DSS and NHS payment, often as well as providing two or three completely free beds (for those not entitled to DSS payment).

There are in excess of 50 treatment centres offering 12-step-based treatment in the UK and Ireland. They all have a history that contains amusing and tragic anecdotes. They all see themselves as struggling against 'the establishment' for recognition and credibility. Some have excellent training programmes and good relationships with local health authorities; all are concerned about future funding and the contract culture.

Controlled research is needed to evaluate these treatment centres, some of which make extravagant claims as part of a marketing strategy. Project Match is viewed as helpful to the 12-step movement.

Some problems

NA is far from perfect. It is a self-help group organised and run by people in varying stages of recovery. Relapse does occur, being treated constructively as a 'learning experience', with individuals being welcomed back.

Some groups are immature, some members are more interested in romantic relationships than recovery, and sometimes bad advice is given, for example by dogmatic individuals who may suggest that drugs such as naltrexone, lithium and disulfiram should be stopped in order to participate in a totally drug-free programme.

Some members describe adverse experience of hospitals and previous help-seeking. Psychiatrists and other professionals are often ridiculed in meetings (sometimes with justification). Mature members, however, in general have a healthy respect for professionals and often make appropriate referrals when things go wrong or problems occur.

Conclusion

NA started in Britain in 1979. It grew rapidly throughout the 1980s/1990s and continues to grow as it develops a good reputation and relationships with professional staff. Whilst there are some problems, it remains an important, freely available adjunct to therapy and after-care for persons and families suffering drug-related problems. Any such clients may usefully be encouraged to attend. Professionals are invited to attend open meetings themselves, many of whom enjoy doing so, often acquiring a list of useful contacts in the process.

NA has much collective wisdom to offer both client and professional. It contains an array of relatively untapped research material and remains a source of energy, enthusiasm, humour and positive feedback to those in the caring professions who deal with problem drinkers and drug takers.

References

Cook, C. (1988). The Minnesota Model in the management of drug and alcohol dependency: miracle, method or myth? Part I: The philosophy and the programme. *British Journal of Addiction*, 83, 625–34. Part II: Evidence and conclusions. *British Journal of Addiction*, 83, 735–48.

NA (Narcotics Anonymous) (1988). *The NA big book*, 5th edn. World Service Office Inc., Van Nuys, CA.

NA (1989). For the newcomer. Information Pamphlet No. 16. UK Service Office, PO Box 704, London SW10.

Robinson, D. (1979). *Talking out of alcoholism*. Croom Helm, London.

Wells, B. (1987). Narcotics Anonymous (NA): the phenomenal growth of an important resource. *British Journal of Addiction*, 82, 581–2.

NB The website for NA in the UK is www.ukna.org

The origins, arrival and spread of residential Minnesota Model centres across the UK

Tim Leighton and Nick Barton

Late in 1974 in Weston-super-Mare, Somerset, a new 'treatment centre' for alcoholics opened in a building previously known as Totterdown Hall. This name presumably being considered unsuitable, it was renamed Broadway Lodge. This was the first of the Minnesota Model centres in Britain, inspired by the American clinics such as Hazelden which had been established in the 1950s.

The impetus for the founding of Broadway came from a small group of business people, members of AA, who wished to provide residential treatment for British alcoholics which had the 12-Step Programme of Alcoholics Anonymous at its core. They sought the help of Hazelden staff to set up a similar programme in the UK.

Origins of the Minnesota Model

By 1950 Alcoholics Anonymous had become established throughout the United States and its philosophy was beginning to be very influential both on public attitudes and on government policy. Moreover a number of individuals who had found recovery in AA were becoming active in setting up and developing agencies to help alcoholics, ranging from night shelters to rehabilitation programmes. In Minnesota in particular, three different programmes were developed in the late 1940s and early 1950s which formed the foundations of what became known as the Minnesota Model. At Willmar State Hospital, the staff invited AA members to become involved in advising and supporting patients, and the decision was made to take alcoholics out of the locked psychiatric wards and give them their own unit. At Pioneer House, a haven for street drinkers was created with a strong basis in the AA philosophy, and at Hazelden a farmhouse was converted to allow a small group of alcoholics 'of the professional class' to live for a few months in an abstinent environment, with a programme of support and education provided by established members of AA (Spicer, 1993).

These programmes achieved a notable measure of success, particularly in contrast to the custodial hospital regimes which had preceded them, and their reputation grew. They attracted the support of local worthies, often in recovery themselves, who provided funds and political support. The staff at Willmar State Hospital, under Nelson Bradley and Daniel Anderson, developed a set of assumptions about alcoholism which were to become the basis of a systematic approach to treatment (see below). Later Dan Anderson moved to Hazelden, which grew into a professional, multi-disciplinary treatment programme. By the mid-1970s it was large (over 100 first-stage beds, an extended care unit and a family centre) and extremely influential. During the late 1970s and the 1980s the Minnesota Model became the dominant approach to treating alcoholism in the United States. The public profile was raised by such figures as Betty Ford, the wife of former President Gerald Ford, who founded her own clinic in California. Many sports and media stars, particularly in the USA, also underwent treatment for alcohol and drug dependence during this period, usually with extensive publicity.

Other drug addictions – the concept of chemical dependence

An important development was when Minnesota Model (MM) treatment centres began to admit those primarily dependent on drugs other than alcohol. It was already recognised that some alcoholics had a propensity to substitute sedatives or tranquillisers for alcohol, and that some users of illicit or prescribed drugs seemed vulnerable to alcohol dependence. The experience of Hazelden and similar clinics was that the same treatment approach was as helpful with drug-addicted people as it was with alcoholics. The notion of Chemical Dependence emerged, and by the time the Minnesota Model arrived in Britain, this condition was what the model was offering to treat. People seeking help with other 'addictive behaviours' such as gambling, and in more recent years compulsive spending, eating and sexual behaviour were also catered for by some, but not all, centres.

Another conceptual development arose from the influence of Family Systems theory. It was observed that families adjusted to an alcohol problem, with each member developing ways of coping. The effect of this was to hinder change, as this would upset the family balance. Minnesota Model centres quickly adopted a focus on the family and social environment of their patients, offering programmes of education and counselling to family members and employers. From this emerged the concepts of the 'family illness' and co-dependency.

What are the elements of the Minnesota Model?

It is difficult to be precise about the elements of a Minnesota programme, as they vary across agencies and have also undergone some development over time. But elements that can usefully be considered are sets of beliefs and

assumptions about the problem, ideas about effective interventions, the therapeutic activities in which clients or patients are engaged, and the nature of
the counselling relationship.

Beliefs and assumptions

According to Dan Anderson, the assumptions about alcoholism, or addiction,
that underpin the model are that it exists, and that it is an illness of some
kind. He describes it as a no-fault illness, that is multiphasic and usually
chronic (Anderson, 1981). There was a strong tendency to view alcoholism
and other addictive illness as primary; in other words, the disruption and
damage to physical and mental health and social relationships were mainly
the result of the addiction rather than the other way around.

Jerry Spicer, until recently President of Hazelden, enumerates three core
perspectives:

- treat people with chemical dependency
- treat them with dignity
- treat them as whole persons – mind, body and spirit.

He contrasts the MM approach with a traditional medical model, and points
out that, in the former, 'patients' are not seen as passive but as active
collaborators in the recovery process. The MM focuses on many areas of
life, expects recovery to be a long-term process rather than a 'cure', is
multidisciplinary, and relies on natural support systems such as the family,
community and self-help groups. It is quite clear from this perspective that
even if no fault or blame is attached to the development of the illness,
alcoholics and drug-dependent people are fully responsible for their recovery
(Spicer, 1993).

12-Step programmes

A major emphasis of Minnesota and related treatment is helping clients to
affiliate with an appropriate 12-Step 'fellowship', usually Alcoholics Anonymous or Narcotics Anonymous. For those whose primary problem is opiates
or other illicit drugs, usually the most suitable programme is Narcotics
Anonymous, whose groups are widely available in many cities of the UK
(for a further account, see Chapter 14, this volume). Narcotics Anonymous,
like AA, is a non-professional organisation, whose philosophy and wisdom
have developed through the experience of its members over the last 50 years.
It is interesting that early in the history of NA, members were quick to
recognise their tendency to substitute one drug for another and their prone-
ness to develop a problematic or addictive relationship with alcohol. The
NA philosophy of complete abstinence from all mood-altering chemicals

including alcohol therefore predates recent research examining, for example, whether the rewarding or anxiety-reducing properties of a variety of drugs with contrasting subjective and psychomotor effects may influence common pathways of neurotransmission.

The 12-Step Programme famously invites addicted people to accept their 'powerlessness' over their addiction, and this has been criticised as encouraging reduced responsibility and self-fulfilling expectancies of failure if a person should lapse back into use. The second point has some force, and most Minnesota Model treatment programmes include a strong element of relapse prevention and lapse management. The first criticism is entirely misguided in our opinion, as the effect of this acceptance is to end years of struggle with self-defeating patterns and usually exhausting and pre-occupying attempts to control and manage the problem. The acceptance of powerlessness is rather like accepting that a relationship has irreparably broken down. Provided support is available, this step lays the foundation for an entirely new way of life. The concept of powerlessness is never intended to serve as an excuse for using or as a way of ducking responsibility.

The other well-known feature of 12-Step recovery is its focus on 'spiritual' recovery, and the invitation to rely on a Higher Power. Again this aspect is open to a great deal of misunderstanding. AA and NA themselves claim that their programmes are 'spiritual not religious', by which they mean not connected to organised or denominational religion. Nevertheless it is pretty clear that for many AA and NA members developing a relationship with 'God', however conceived of, is in fact a 'religious' undertaking in an ordinary sense. However, as some observers and researchers have pointed out (e.g. Ken Hart), 12-Step recovery comes in two distinct flavours, one plainly 'religious' and the other entirely secular (Hart, 1999). For the latter, the 'Higher Power' may consist in a set of values, or the collective wisdom of the group. The 12-Step Programme, with its emphasis on personal inventory and mending damaged relationships, may offer a more or less existentialist opportunity to live authentically or 'in good faith'. The point is that recovery must have personal meaning, of a sustainable and developing kind. A programme offering a more meaningful life has great appeal for many addicted people, particularly those who are demoralised and whose self-esteem has been damaged. A recent British study showed that, in a non-12-Step NHS substance misuse unit in London, many of the clients were attracted to the 12-Step Programme, but they tended to approve of or agree with those steps which stress responsibility and making amends, and to dislike those which overtly mentioned God or prayer (Best et al., 2001; Harris et al., 2002).

Another obvious advantage of AA and NA is the availability of a supportive group of people, outside the family system, who are dedicated to helping each other stay abstinent. Much research into the maintenance of change has supported the idea that social support for change is as important or more important than any internal psychological factors. Minnesota Model treatment lays great stress on the notion of people with similar problems helping each other, and the great majority of the structured activity in treatment consists of mutually helpful group work.

Moreover if it is accepted that the family or social system of the addicted person has adapted to the addiction problem, in order to cope with it, or because its presence might serve some useful function for the system, then for some time at least there may be forces in that system tending towards or inviting relapse. If a recovering person joins a mutual-support group which fosters recovering attitudes and behaviour, and provides a structure and rationale for change, this can serve as an antidote to such pressures, and at the same time allow the person to remain connected to their family and friends. If recovery is sustained, the system will in time adapt to the new situation, and this can be made more likely if support and help for the necessary adjustments are offered to family members and intimate friends. There are similar self-help fellowships available such as Families Anonymous for family members. Minnesota Model centres share an agreement that affiliation with AA or NA, etc., is usually a very important contribution to sustained recovery, and place emphasis on facilitating such affiliation for clients and their family members.

The British context

The arrival of the Minnesota Model in the UK, and its establishment as a professional and ever more respected approach to the treatment of addiction, occurred in the context of much pioneering work by clinicians such as Max Glatt, who for several decades advocated, in an intelligent, humane and unfanatical way, the usefulness of AA and the 'disease concept' in alcoholism treatment. The idea that the Minnesota Model brought the true revelation of the 'disease concept' to the woad-besmeared Britons is quite incorrect. The treatment of alcoholism and drug addiction was thoroughly 'medicalised' throughout the 1960s and 1970s, both within the NHS and the private sector. Many of the regimes in the Alcoholism Treatment Units set up in each region during the 1960s contained elements such as opportunities to attend AA meetings, stress on abstinence as a treatment goal and so on, which are characteristic of the MM. Glatt's treatment programme at Warlingham Park and the units at St Bernard's (Ealing, West London) and at many other hospitals are clearly cousins of the American approach.

It is interesting that at around the same time as the Minnesota Model was arriving, the old disease concept was falling into disrepute in Europe, with two different influences aiding that process. One was the concept of the Dependence Syndrome, and the other was the challenge presented by psychologists and others, some of whom formed the New Directions in Alcohol Group precisely to question the medical model and the absolutist insistence on abstinence as the only proper treatment goal. We would like to think that after a period of mutual ignorance, followed by a variety of uncomprehending stand-offs, that both of these strands have had a profound influence on the philosophy and programme design of the leading Minnesota Model agencies in Britain.

What was new when Broadway Lodge opened in 1974 was the concentration of the programme: it involved a considerably shorter stay than the typical Alcohol Treatment Unit (ATU) (6–8 weeks rather than 3 months or more) and the detoxification and medical services were integrated with the psychosocial treatment in a more coherent way. The 12-Step component became a core element rather than an add-on. There was more stress laid on the peer group as the primary agent of change and support. And later of course people addicted to other drugs, including opiates, began to be admitted.

The Minnesota Model has usually been offered in the private sector, and several units were established in the 1980s and 1990s by private hospital groups. However, following Broadway Lodge, several centres such as Clouds House in Wiltshire, Broadreach House in Devon and the Chemical Dependency Centre in London, were established as non-profit charitable agencies, whose aim was to serve a much broader social spectrum. Since its foundation in 1983, Clouds House has always had a majority of state-funded clients, originally through the DHSS, but later through Local Health Authorities, Social Services Community Care funds, Probation money or a combination of these (Georgakis, 1995). This has meant that in the charitable treatment units there has always been an exciting and broad social mix. Some of these clients have very severe problems, but it has been found that many of them benefit from this model of treatment as well.

The treatment

Interventions

The treatment at Hazelden has always been multimodal, and this applies to most UK centres too. It has never consisted of a pure 12-Step facilitation model as developed for Project MATCH. For example in the late 1970s psychologists at Hazelden began to use Rational Emotive Therapy to help patients deal with emotional states regarded as risky for relapse. Glasser's Reality Therapy was also influential. An individual treatment plan is developed from a comprehensive assessment, which hopes to address those issues which have a bearing on the maintenance of abstinence and a more satisfying lifestyle. The focus might be on interpersonal difficulties, feelings management, social skills, spiritual development, or use of leisure time, and a patient typically works on a manageable range of these. The individualised elements are overlaid on a basis consisting of education about addiction and a firm recommendation to become involved in the 12-Step fellowships of AA or NA.

The treatment programme consists of daily group therapy, individual counselling sessions, educational lectures, workshops and reading, together with individual written assignments focusing on the issues in the treatment plan. If possible, family or couple conferences may be held to encourage a cohesive approach to the problem and to discuss expectations for the future. Some agencies offer relaxation techniques, education in leisure, exercise and nutrition, and may have alternative therapies such as acupuncture available. The so-called first-stage residential treatment centres usually have full medical detoxification facilities, and physical recuperation is also attended to by the medical staff.

Counselling style

The Minnesota Model developed a reputation for a highly confrontational counselling style that some might describe as brutal or even abusive. Yet many counsellors working within the model as it is practised in the UK today would not recognise this description. One of the central tenets of the model is 'treat people with chemical dependence with dignity'. So where does this reputation come from and is there any basis to it? There is no doubt that in some agencies both in the USA and in Britain there is still a risk that clients may be exposed to a coercive, pressurising approach. However, this is not at all in the true spirit of the model, and there is no evidence that it is effective. Such an approach is unacceptable. In the mid-1970s when the model was introduced into Britain there were certain ideas very prominent in the addictions field, for example that an addicted person had to be 'broken down' in order to be rebuilt with different, more responsible attitudes and behaviours. From a disease model perspective, 'denial' was seen as a crucial symptom of addiction and that sufferers needed to be relentlessly challenged, preferably by alcoholic peers who would 'see through the denial', in order to defeat it. The favoured approach to confronting denial today is a gentler, respectful one, which assumes that if a person feels safe and if their personal dignity and autonomy are not too threatened, they will be less defensive.

The predominant style remains active, focused and directive, and most MM counsellors will attempt to inculcate a fairly clear-cut, simple idea of addiction based on a 12-Step formulation. The approach is profoundly pragmatic: the scientific respectability of a concept or idea is less important than whether it is effective in mobilising behaviours which are believed to be necessary to initiate and maintain abstinent recovery. Counsellors often have an eclectic style, integrating a Motivational Enhancement approach, or techniques borrowed from Cognitive Therapy. At Clouds House, for example, team supervision includes the use of Diagrammatic Reformulation derived from Cognitive Analytic Therapy (CAT) (Ryle, 1995).

The main task of the counsellor is to help the client focus on the treatment plan, to exhort and educate, and to facilitate involvement in a support network, whose main element will be AA or NA. The counsellor should help the client make use of group therapy and participation in the residential community to explore their interpersonal patterns and relate these to potential pitfalls in recovery.

Who can benefit?

Conventional wisdom had it that this particular model was only suitable for those from reasonably stable middle-class backgrounds and perhaps where there was at least some vestige of a Christian-based value system. However, research into the outcomes of Clouds House and the subsequent findings of the National Treatment Outcome Research Study (NTORS) indicated that the model can be successfully applied to people from disadvantaged backgrounds as well. Although there is no specific research yet available there is at least anecdotal evidence that the model can benefit those from a variety of ethnic and religious contexts.

A changing population

Over the years there has been a marked decline in the numbers of older alcohol-dependent people finding their way to the 12-Step residential treatment centres. This has been due partly to the drop in the state funding available to those seeking treatment for alcohol dependency via Community Care and the tidal shift in government policy towards a concentration upon drug treatment driven by a desire to reduce crime. Overall the average age of those being admitted is falling, possibly because they are starting their substance-misusing careers earlier and are being picked up sooner by a more responsive system.

There is no doubt that the change in cultural norms where drug use is concerned poses problems for total abstinence programmes. The safety valve provided by acceptance of a personal vulnerability to 'cross-addiction' may be more and more challenged by those seeking to be selective about their use. Research is needed about the acceptability to clients of complete abstinence, but actually the advisability of such a course does not seem to be such a commonly expressed stumbling block as one might expect.

The usefulness of a 'disease concept' is also attenuated these days, as many of our clients have had obviously difficult and traumatic lives and grew up in a drug-rich environment, and it is clear that many initiated regular drug use as a way of coping. However, the traditional model of treating or addressing the 'underlying issues' and seeing addiction purely as a symptom of dysfunctional coping or disordered personality risks minimising the impact of the addiction in creating problems, perpetuating them and making them worse. The reasons why a person initiates a behaviour may be quite different from what maintains that behaviour, and most people who use drugs and alcohol to 'cope' do not develop chronic addiction problems. As far as the disease concept is concerned, it does not appear to be an essential pillar of the 12-Step philosophy, at least in the culture of the UK. Interesting research by Christo and Franey (1995) showed that around half of a sample of British NA members with a good foundation of abstinent recovery did not regard their addiction as a 'disease'.

Because residential treatment is comparatively expensive, only the more severely dependent people or those with complex social and psychological profiles are now gaining access to such treatment. The exceptions are those who can pay privately or who have medical insurance. This has both favourable and unfavourable effects. The drastic nature of residential treatment and the stringency of the complete abstinence goal are most suitable for those with severe dependence and a substantial period of problematic use. The philosophy often makes more sense to them and there has been time for a history of seriously negative consequences to accrue. However, those with severe and complex problems need more support and more skilful intervention, and have a greater tendency to discharge themselves from treatment or behave in ways leading to being discharged. They are often seriously demoralised and anxious and may be suffering from depression or other psychiatric disorders. They usually need continuing support and therefore need sustained funding to cover this.

New settings

Most of the Minnesota Model centres offer short-stay residential programmes. The residential setting allows for the integration of detoxification and medical services, gives respite from the chaos and problems of life outside, and offers a concentrated group and community experience in which the maximum dose of therapeutic learning can be administered. The short stay prevents institutionalisation, and allows the client to return to their families and jobs relatively quickly, properly prepared to tackle the challenges of recovery.

On the other hand, for other clients, more benefit will result from extended involvement in a counselling or support programme which may be residential, a structured day programme or weekly aftercare counselling, individually or in a group.

There has also been a move towards offering first-stage (post-detox) treatment in a non-residential structured day setting, and many agencies including Clouds run such day programmes. The treatment tasks and activities are very similar to those in residential settings. Although research evidence from the USA shows little difference in outcomes for uncomplicated alcohol dependent clients between residential and non-residential treatment, it is far from clear that this applies to drug-dependent clients or those with dual diagnoses or complex problems. It seems as though some of these may do better with the additional structure and containment of a residential setting, and there is certainly evidence that for drug-dependent clients, involvement in some level of counselling or treatment for an extended period is associated with better outcomes. The optimum is to provide what a person needs and no more, and the intensity of treatment setting and support should reduce as the person becomes able to function more independently.

Residential treatment of another sort has also appeared with the 12-Step-based programme of the Rehabilitation of Addicted Prisoners Trust (RAPT) achieving interesting results within some of Her Majesty's most secure accommodation.

Development of the model

The singular, standardised approach that relied heavily on daily inculcation of the principles enshrined in the 12 steps has given way to a more broadly based intervention. Naturally there are still centres that are more traditionalist than others. However, whereas there had once been a tendency to assume invariably that if the treatment was unsuccessful with a particular person it had more to do with the individual's state of readiness or approach to treatment than it did with the treatment itself, there is a greater willingness to question received wisdom. Perhaps because so many charitable organisations are involved there is an awareness of the need to help as many as possible. This, amongst other things, has led to an increasing responsiveness to individuals and a growing flexibility of approach.

In the early days treatment and care staff were almost invariably drawn from the ranks of those who were themselves in recovery. It was thought that only they could truly understand the predicament of patients as well as being able to serve as living examples of recovery. They often took the role of salaried versions of the anonymous fellowship sponsors. There is still a high proportion amongst those working in such services as counsellors but this has been evened out somewhat by those not in recovery. The work nonetheless attracts many people whose families have experienced some sort of substance-related problem.

While 'working the steps' and external attendance at AA or NA meetings remain essential elements of the treatment programme much more attention is now paid to ambivalence, motivation for change, interpersonal relationships, family involvement, relapse prevention and onward referral than was originally the case. There has been an integration of the 12-Step core with cognitive behavioural interventions. Cognitive Analytic Therapy has also been found to have a compatible application in some centres (Ryle, 1995).

The future – adaptation and evolution

In an interesting interview in 1992, Dan Anderson, one of the originators of the 'Minnesota Model' in the 1950s and a modest and pragmatic man, said:

Everybody thinks I should go around defending the Minnesota Model. But when Bradley and I developed it, it was a temporary thing. We never thought it would last. And the show has had too long a run, really, I say. I don't care what you replace it with; do anything that works. That's what we did in the first place. I mean, I have no sacred investment in the model.

(Spicer, 1993)

Those who adopted the Minnesota Model in the UK did so with the fervour of true believers, which of course stifled any impulse to objective examination. Centres attracted such a volume of referrals throughout the 1980s that there was little incentive to find out whether the approach was indeed producing the benefit claimed. But major developments have now taken place, as described above, and have taken the treatment model quite a long way from its origins. The model is being applied in day programme and other settings as well as in residential. There is more openness to influence from other approaches, and a more coherent integration of these is taking place, improving on a tendency to amateur eclecticism. Some of the conceptual pillars which originally supported the model have been found to be unnecessary and have been dismantled. Treatment centres are serving a broader constituency than previously.

Today, in the UK, there is a growing interest in and respect for the 12-Step approach, from clients, care managers, commissioners of treatment and even academic researchers. The NTORS study found treatment to be generally effective both in the community and in residential programmes. In reports from NTORS reporting on follow-up of clients from residential rehabilitation (Gossop et al., 1999; Stewart et al., 2000), the observation is made that 'the clients in the residential programmes presented with some of the most severe problems and complex needs, and these clients made some of the greatest treatment gains'.

The battle over abstinence has cooled. The place of abstinence as a sensible and achievable goal for severely dependent clients is recognised, as is the value of harm reduction strategies and moderation goals for some clients. As treatment agencies in this tradition grow and develop, they will continue to have a significant part to play in the management of Britain's substance misuse problem. In particular the attention paid to alcohol as a serious contributor to the problems of drug users, the management of impaired and dually diagnosed patients in intensive, multi-disciplinary residential programmes, and the focus on providing help and support to families as well as to the drug users, will all be areas in which this tradition can continue to make a vital contribution in the twenty-first century.

References

Anderson, D. J. (1981). *Perspectives on Treatment: The Minnesota Experience*, Center City, MN: Hazelden.

Best, D., Harris, J., Gossop, M., Manning, V., Man, L., Marshall, J., Bearn, J. and Strang, J. (2001). Are the 12 Steps more acceptable to drug users than to drinkers? *European Addiction Research*, 7: 69–77.

Christo, G. and Franey, C. (1995). Drug users' spiritual beliefs, locus of control, and the disease concept in relation to Narcotics Anonymous attendance and six-month outcomes. *Drug and Alcohol Dependence*, 38: 51–56.

Georgakis, A. (1995). *Evaluation of a Residential Alcohol and Drug Dependency Treatment Centre* (privately published by Clouds).

Gossop, M., Marsden, J., Stewart, D. and Rolfe, A. (1999). Treatment retention and one-year outcomes for residential programmes in England. *Drug and Alcohol Dependence*, 57: 89–98.

Harris, J., Best, D., Gossop, M., Marshall, J., Man, L.-H., Manning, V. and Strang, J. (2002). Prior Alcoholics Anonymous (AA) affiliation and the acceptability of the twelve steps to patients entering UK statutory addiction treatment. *Journal of Studies on Alcohol*, 64: 257–61.

Hart, K. (1999). A spiritual interpretation of the 12-steps of Alcoholics Anonymous: from resentment to forgiveness to love. *Journal of Ministry in Addiction and Recovery*, 6(2): 25–39.

Ryle, A. (ed.) (1995). *Cognitive Analytic Therapy: Developments in Theory and Practice*, Chichester: John Wiley.

Spicer, J. (1993). *The Minnesota Model: The Evolution of the Multidisciplinary Approach to Addiction Recovery*, Center City, MN: Hazelden.

Stewart, D., Gossop, M., Marsden, J. and Treacy, S. (2000). Variation between and within drug treatment modalities: data from the National Treatment Outcome Research Study (NTORS), UK. *European Addiction Research*, 6: 106–114.

Chapter 16

Treatment to order

The new drug treatment and testing orders

Emily Finch and Mike Ashton

The 1998 Crime and Disorder Bill introduced 'Drug Treatment and Testing Orders' (DTTOs) as an innovative sentencing option for drug-misusing offenders, with the clear stated objective of reducing the crime associated with drug misuse. However, the DTTO is, in reality, the product of a process of development in drug and sentencing policy in the UK which has been going on throughout the last 30 years. So far there is limited evidence as to their effectiveness, but they are already having a substantial impact on local service planning and policy.

The reason for the interest

Addiction to cocaine and heroin (and to a lesser extent some other drugs) is clearly associated with a marked increase in acquisitive crime. Furthermore, the successful treatment of this addiction reduces crime, and treatment for some particular types of drug misuse, especially methadone maintenance for opiate misuse, has been shown repeatedly to be effective in reducing crime. In the UK National Treatment Outcome Research Study (NTORS), 753 clients were followed up for one year after recruitment to various treatment modalities. Over the year the number of crimes committed was reduced to about one-third of intake levels and the amount of criminal involvement was reduced to a half (Gossop *et al.* 2000). Ball and Ross (1991) found that there were major reductions in crimes committed to fund drug use in a population of opiate-addicted individuals treated in methadone programmes on the east coast of the United States. The number of crimes committed fell to 20 per cent of pre-treatment levels. Other long-term follow-up studies of drug users in treatment in the USA and Australia have shown that crime is reduced consistently in those individuals who are retained in methadone treatment (Hubbard *et al.* 1989; Simpson 1990; Bell *et al.* 1992). However, a meta-analysis of treatment outcome confirmed that methadone mainten-ance reduced crime but with a wide variation in effect size and some studies showing no significant reductions. It is suggested that the largest changes are seen in studies which measure drug-related and property crime and less change seen in crime which may not be associated with drug use (Grapendaal *et al.* 1994; Marsch 1998).

Recent joint treatment-control developments

Since the 1970s there has been a legal framework which has allowed drug misusers to be diverted from the criminal justice system into treatment. Various Criminal Justice Acts have allowed treatment for drug problems as a condition of a probation order, although there were always problems in funding these episodes of treatment.

Schedule 1A 6 of the 1991 Criminal Justice Act allowed drug misusers to be referred for treatment as a condition of a probation order. Initially these orders were used very little for individual offenders but towards the middle of the 1990s local initiatives began to be encouraged.

All over the United Kingdom locally planned and funded projects were set up which used the 1991 legislation. Most involve some sort of intensive supervision on a probation order provided in partnership with local agencies. The 'CRISP' project (Community Rehabilitation and Intensive Supervision Project) in Bromley had offenders managed by the local non-statutory sector drug agency in partnership with probation, with some supervision from the local police. Another project run in East Kent similarly provides a high level of community supervision in conjunction with treatment.

The 'STEP' project in Wakefield has been modelled on drug courts which have been extensively used in the USA. A designated court 'sentences' an offender to treatment, provided by a local drug agency and imposes certain conditions on that offender. The court then reviews the offender regularly and re-sentences them if necessary.

In the 1990s explicit partnerships between criminal justice and health were set up with the publication of 'Tackling Drugs Together' in 1995, which set out government drug strategy for England (with Scotland, Wales and Northern Ireland having their own strategies). Criminal justice and health-related issues were given equal emphasis and clear goals were given for both. It set up Drug Action Teams in all parts of the country which had chief officer representation from the police, health and social service purchasers. In 1997 the New Labour government continued this strategy with its strong emphasis on partnership. The appointment of an ex-policemen as the UK anti-drug coordinator gave the clear message that criminal justice had a pivotal role to play in the control of the drug misuse problem. 'Tackling Drugs to Build a Better Britain', a ten-year drug strategy published in 1998, reinforced a policy which encompassed education, control of drug supply and treatment.

Legal aspects of Drug Treatment and Testing Orders

Drug Treatment and Testing orders (DTTOs) were a key component of the Crime and Disorder Act 1998. The rationale for their introduction includes the evidence described above that drug misuse is linked to crime, that coercive treatment enforced through the criminal justice system is at least as effective as non-coerced treatment and that there is good evidence from the UK that treatment does indeed reduce drug use.

The drug treatment and testing order is a community sentence in its own right and is administered by probation services. Its objective is to encourage convicted drug users to enter treatment as an alternative to other sentencing options, including prison. The treatment is commissioned at a local level by providers specifically contracted to do so or in some cases directly by the DTTO team. The testing component of the order requires the individual user to provide specimens for drug testing and that those results will be available to the court.

The orders can be made in magistrates' or crown courts only if arrangements have been specifically made for service provision in an area. Orders can be made for between six months and three years. Clients can only be made subject to an order if they are assessed to be 'dependent on or has a propensity to misuse drugs' and if 'his dependency or propensity is such as requires and may be susceptible to treatment'. The Act contains specific requirements for testing – 'the court may, by order, require him to provide samples of such a description as it may specify'. The court has to be satisfied that arrangements have been made for the treatment to be provided. For the duration of the order a client is under the supervision of a probation officer who is required to report the client's progress to the court responsible for the order. The order is reviewed at intervals of not less than one month and a report has to be given to the court before each review. The court then has powers to continue with the order, to amend the order or to revoke the order.

Clinical aspects of Drug Treatment and Testing Orders

The treatment provided in the context of Drug Treatment and Testing Orders can under the terms of the Act take many forms. It is intended to be customised to meet the individual's needs and may include the full range of treatment options including residential rehabilitation, inpatient and outpatient detoxification, day programmes, methadone maintenance and individual counselling sessions. The three initial pilot Drug Treatment and Testing Order schemes were located in three deliberately very different parts of England – Croydon (Surrey), Gloucestershire and Liverpool. DTTO programmes vary substantially in the treatment they offer although the programme implemented in the Croydon pilot has been fully described (Ashton 2001; Finch et al. 2003). There, a designated team of probation officers and nurses acted as case workers and supervising officers. Following assessment a treatment plan was devised for each client. This was presented to court. Options available included inpatient detoxification from opiates using methadone, lofexidine or naltrexone or from cocaine using antidepressants where indicated. Some clients then went on to residential rehabilitation. Clients can be prescribed methadone on a reduction or maintenance basis. All clients in the community attended a day programme three days a week involving protocol-driven relapse prevention, reasoning and rehabilitation and schema-focused therapy. Motivational enhancement and crisis resolution work was done by key workers in individual sessions.

Ethical issues in DTTOs

At its extreme, opposition to coerced treatment is fundamental, and indeed Thomas Szasz regards drug use as voluntary and therefore by definition not requiring treatment (Szasz 1982). However, many other potential ethical issues arise when managing coerced clients and need to be considered before DTTO programmes can be implemented.

It is potentially unethical to force clients into treatment choices at all. Indeed many professionals in the field of treatment for drug misusers regard any form of coercion as an anathema and believe that clients will only do well in treatment if they have chosen to have it for themselves. This belief, however, is not supported by research evidence which would indicate that clients in coerced treatment do as well as those in non-coerced treatment. The nature of coercion is complex and many other non-criminal justice pressures are perceived as coercive. Within DTTOs subjects are offered a range of treatments and do have a choice of which treatment modality they want to enter.

Treatment which is offered under the criminal justice coercion needs to be effective. It would be unethical to coerce individuals into a form of treatment when research evidence has shown that another form of treatment is more effective. It is also important to ensure that treatment expectations are not too great. This may be especially true when partnerships between probation and treatment providers are set up. Probation may have high expectations of treatment which may in many cases be impossible to achieve. For instance, total abstinence from all substances may be expected from clients despite a treatment agency's clinical experience which would predict that some clients may achieve good outcomes on long-term substitute prescriptions.

Queue jumping is likely to be a difficult issue both nationally and locally. In many areas of the UK, treatment for opiate users is effectively rationed with waiting lists for both outpatient and inpatient treatment and very few places available for residential rehabilitation. Offenders who are given DTTOs may be able to receive treatment immediately and indeed may receive better quality more intensive treatment than non-offenders. It is possible that this may become politically unacceptable.

Are DTTOs effective?

The three pilot schemes were evaluated by Turnbull *et al.* (2000). In each area special teams consisting of probation officers and health and drug worker staff assessed offenders referred to them and decided whether to propose a drug treatment and testing order to the court. From 554 referrals, 288 proposals were made resulting in 210 orders.

Interviews with 132 offenders shortly after they started their orders revealed that despite long and intense drug-using careers, three-fifths had never received formal help for their drug problems. Typically they were young white men unemployed for several years and heavily into drugs and drug-taking circles. They averaged 31 previous convictions and four in five had been in prison, on average five times. Acquisitive crime accounted for the vast majority's current sentence. Before arrest, 91 per cent had been using heroin daily (of whom three-fifths were injecting) and three-quarters were using crack. A typical weekly drug spend of £400 was funded mainly through shoplifting, burglary and selling drugs.

Half the offenders on the orders were either detoxified or placed on a reducing prescription and a third in residential rehabilitation. Though over 90 per cent were opiate addicts, just a fifth received maintenance treatment. There were clear differences in treatment philosophy between the three pilot sites with Gloucester insisting on early abstinence and Croydon and Liverpool expecting offenders to progress only slowly towards abstinence, a difference reflected in treatment dispositions: two-thirds of the offenders in Croydon received maintenance but none in Gloucestershire. Typically orders were made for 12 months, though in Croydon nearly half were for 18 months or longer, possibly reflecting Croydon's preference for the maintenance option.

The intention that the sentencing court would remain responsible for reviewing the offender's progress was achieved in four out of five review hearings in Liverpool but in only a third and fifth of cases at the other two sites. Arrangements in Liverpool were aided by the dedication of a set time to the hearings and arranging for them to be heard mainly by one of two magistrates. Across the three sites, reviews averaged nine minutes to complete and were usually monthly. In 8 out of 10 cases the court did not amend the order but staff did see reviews as important motivators for the offender.

Eligibility for a DTTO entails eligibility for a community sentence, but its targeting at persistent high-rate offenders means that many may have otherwise been imprisoned. Sentencers reported that, as intended, in many cases the testing element of the order gave them the confidence to use it when otherwise they would have delivered a custodial sentence. When an order is revoked the offender is re-sentenced for the original offence. At least two-thirds then received a custodial sentence, confirming that the orders did act as an alternative to imprisonment.

Interviews with three different samples of offenders placed on the orders were the main means for determining their effectiveness. One sample had been on the order for about six weeks, another six months. 'Exit' interviews were conducted with a third sample who were either nearing the end of their order or had come out the other end (completed or revoked). In each case, current crime and drug use were compared with the same individuals' activities before arrest. The samples must have overlapped but were not simply the same people at different times. This is why they present slightly different profiles even when the figures refer to the same point in time, such as before their arrest. Broadly, while on the order, the responses given by the offenders indicate that they have dramatically cut their drug use and crime, but the former is only partially confirmed by test data and there remains a very large gap in the data: at the three stages, between a third and two-thirds of prisoners had either dropped out of contact or had been thrown off the order so were not interviewed. Overwhelmingly the results came from people *still actively participating in their order*.

Early progress

Of the 210 offenders placed on orders, 132 attended the schemes long enough to be interviewed about six weeks into their orders. As already noted, broadly they matched the profile of the more criminally active clients seen by drug treatment services, but most had never before been in treatment. After this short time on the order, the proportion using heroin in the past four weeks had fallen by 30 per cent and the proportion using crack by 35 per cent. From typically spending £400 a week buying illicit drugs, a third were no longer in this market and the typical drug spend of the remainder had fallen to £70. Since starting their orders, two-thirds had stopped committing acquisitive crime and a further fifth had reduced their offending: in the month before their arrest, 119 offenders had committed on average 137 acquisitive crimes each. After six weeks on the order the 35 still offending averaged 34 crimes each. Interviewees who reported selling drugs also fell by almost two-thirds from 29 to 11.

Mid-term

After six months on their orders, 48 offenders (about 70 per cent of those who had reached this point without their order being revoked) were interviewed. They were generally satisfied with all aspects of the process and had built on the progress made earlier. Though just 19 were drug-free, most felt being on the order had helped them stop (30) or reduce (17) their use of illicit drugs. In the past month just 15 had used heroin and five cocaine or crack, three-quarters who had been injecting before arrest had stopped, and just one (compared to the majority before arrest) had shared injecting equipment or paraphernalia. They felt helped by the structure and intensity of the programmes, support from staff, and access to detoxification and residential rehabilitation services. Nineteen were still buying illicit drugs but typically spending just £50 a week. Only a few were still committing revenue-raising crimes (three selling drugs, one fraud, three shoplifting).

Exit

'Exit' interviews were conducted with 31 offenders who had completed or nearly completed their orders. Between them they had committed over 3,000 acquisitive crimes in the month before their arrest. Now all said they were no longer committing acquisitive crimes and all but four said they were no longer using illicit drugs apart from cannabis. Weekly spending on illicit drugs for the nine continuing to purchase averaged just £28. If their claims are valid, these 31 subjects (or more precisely, the five who had actually completed their orders) represent the schemes' successful 'graduates'. Another 19 offenders whose orders had been revoked were interviewed on average eight months later. Compared to the time when they were subject to the order, they tended to have increased their drug use and crime but both remained far lower than before their arrest. Five (down from 11) were still using crack and 12 (down from 18) heroin, but their weekly drug spend was typically £53 rather than £420. An average monthly tally of 190 acquisitive crimes before arrest had fallen to 48.

Testing results

Urine tests required by the orders provide only a partial check on the validity of the offenders' reports. Such tests do not reflect *reductions* in drug use unless these are great enough for blood levels to fall below the threshold for triggering a positive result. Over the course of the study, results were available for 2,555 tests from 173 of the offenders. Over 4 in 10 were positive for opiates and about the same proportion for cocaine. Only in Liverpool did the proportion of urine tests positive for cocaine fall as offenders progressed through their orders, but on the face of it the results for opiates were more positive. In the first four weeks of their orders, 128 out of 157 tested offenders provided urines positive for opiates, typically two to three times. But as offenders progressed through their orders the proportion of tests positive for opiates fell from over half to under a third at around the mid-term. In contrast, the rate of cocaine positives remained high, largely due to persistent high rates in Croydon of around 50–60 per cent.

However, the drop in the proportion of opiate-positive tests might have been due to the winnowing out of those who continued to use these drugs.

Offenders who persisted in pre-arrest patterns of opiate use are also the ones most likely to have been left out of the dataset because they were not tested due to revocation of their orders, failure to attend for testing, and/or reconviction for further offending. If this was the case, the drop cannot be considered an indicator of success, rather that 'failures' were diverted out of the schemes. Also the baseline from which improvement was measured was contaminated by the inclusion of tests actually done before the order started. The net result is that even with respect to opiates we cannot be sure that over the entire intake to the schemes the proportion of offenders testing positive did actually fall.

Failure to comply with the order was common, usually in the form of not attending for treatment or supervision or continued use of illicit drugs, especially near the start of the order. By the end of the study, 96 orders (46 per cent of the 210 made) had been revoked, a proportion which was bound to rise further as offenders continued on orders beyond the end of the study. Revocations by the court follow an unacceptable failure to comply on the part of the offender. The high revocation rate across the three sites is largely due to the 60 per cent rate in Gloucestershire, where the project initially insisted on offenders becoming drug-free within two weeks (later extended to six to eight weeks) without the support of maintenance prescribing or a methadone prescription, and where long distances and travel times made it harder for offenders to keep appointments. In Liverpool, just 28 per cent of orders were revoked. Breach proceedings were mainly initiated for failure to attend for appointments rather than positive tests. At two of the sites offenders had to attend appointments at least daily every weekday, but in Liverpool intensity of contact was set individually and may have been just weekly (though attendance for treatment might have been more regular). At the same site urine testing was once a week or less, compared to several times a week at the other sites.

Partnership

This combination of health, drug worker and probation staff working in a criminal justice context is not new, but the DTTO pilots were the first time that such togetherness had been imposed by government. Clashing professional traditions and values were a serious obstacle to the inter-agency working integral to the success of the schemes and contributed to 'considerable conflict' at one scheme, where the quality of the work suffered, and high staff turnover at another which derailed initial plans. A recurring issue was how to engender understanding and respect for the different disciplines' methods and goals without duplicating roles, unrealistically wasteful both in time and in the failure to exploit each member's special skills. However, one of the schemes showed that many of the issues could be resolved at least sufficiently to build an effective team. That site was characterised by a professional attitude from high-calibre leadership and staff, active engagement with the issues with sufficient management time devoted to their resolution, and regular and professionally conducted liaison meetings between lead agencies which were prepared to devolve responsibility for operational matters to the team's leader.

What do these results mean?

To dent the national burden of drug-related crime and make their contribution to achieving national targets, DTTO schemes must process a substantial proportion of high-rate drug-driven offenders. There is evidence from the pilots that they might be able to meet this criterion. Although they may only be able to process 5,000 offenders per year, this figure is significant as nationally only about 1 in 10 of the 200,000 dependent heroin/cocaine users in the UK are high-rate offenders (Gossop *et al.* 2000). DTTOs may therefore be able to reach a significant proportion of these.

Do they save more than they cost? Cost–savings estimates derived from NTORS suggest that just 3,008 offenders would need to have been processed by the schemes in a year in order to cover their costs, well within the intended capacity and within the capacity indicated by the study.

Are they better than the alternatives? Without a comparison group processed normally through the probation options, prisons and treatment services of a pre-DTTO system it can only be assumed that offenders did better than they would have done in conventional treatment. Standard probation orders, and treatment orders without a testing requirement, are also associated with reductions in offending and drug use of the same order of magnitude as seen on the new orders. However, many offenders placed on drug treatment and testing orders would not have been given the chance of a standard probation order by sentencers for whom testing lends credibility to the new order.

There were many gaps in the data from the pilot evaluation. Baseline data for behaviour before the orders was not collected at the time but reconstructed by interviewing offenders whilst they were on the orders. The only data which indicated that progress was made was reported by the offenders themselves; some may have been wary about admitting to continuing crime. These factors make the results from the evaluation less reliable and a shaky foundation for the national policy roll-out which was based on the pilot's interim findings.

The future

There are many potential problems when DTTO programmes are introduced. Inevitably the implementation of DTTOs will require partnerships with different agencies working closely with each other. Expectations of treatment may be different within these agencies and these beliefs need to be expressed and agreed outcomes must be defined before a programme is set up. Sanctions which will be operated if any offender fails to comply again need to be defined and agreed. Treatment programmes need to decide what boundaries they place on offenders especially concerning such issues as failing to attend appointments. Relationships which allow good liaison between agencies are important both in the key local agencies involved and in many other local organisations such as the local police and primary care. Staff teams need to be assembled carefully with good cohesive management both clinically and around the criminal justice input. Professional roles may need to be carefully explored with clear guidelines for which tasks are appropriate for which professional group.

Medical input will be needed in any DTTO programme involving pre-scribing or management of drug users with severe drug problems or associated psychiatric symptoms. Guidance needs to be given which recognises the research evidence that most heroin addicts do better in maintenance pro-grammes (Sees *et al.* 2000). Training for all professionals will be needed and it may be that an expansion of DTTOs nationwide will result in shortages of appropriately trained staff. There will also be the huge challenge of treating large numbers of crack users (many also dependent on heroin) who get picked up by the criminal justice system and who without this coercion would not previously have entered treatment.

In the future, probation services will have to make decisions about the types of treatment they commission for offenders who are given DTTOs. Various factors are important (Rotgers 1992). First, a broad range of treat-ment options need to be available to allow for the best chance of successful treatment outcome. In general all clients need to be offered the same range of treatment options so they can make informed choices about their treatment and so decisions are not made on grounds other than clinical need. Both these factors imply that funding needs to be adequate to allow this broad range of treatment to be available. Decisions regarding the exact nature of treatment need to be made on professional rather than criminal justice grounds. The goals of coercion (i.e. what outcomes are expected) must be reasonably well defined and the results of non-compliance need to be clear. Treatment agencies and criminal justice services need to clarify the nature of their relationship and the expected outcomes. This needs to be communicated to the client. Issues such as confidentiality, frequency of urine testing and consequences of the results need to be understood. Routine evaluation of programme outcomes and research into the optimal ways of managing clients on DTTOs must continue.

Finally, DTTOs have been conceived by politicians looking for an answer to the problem of drug-related crime. Their implementation and functioning needs to be done making maximum use of the evidence generated by pilot studies and previous research on coerced treatment. New evidence needs to be gathered which will allow their effectiveness to be reliably evaluated. Only then will both individual offenders and society benefit.

References

Ashton, M. (2001). First test for the DTTO. *Drug and Alcohol Findings*, 6, 16–21.

Bell, J., Hall, W. and Byth, K. (1992). Changes in criminal activity after entering methadone maintenance. *British Journal of Addiction*, 87, 251–258.

Finch, E., Brotchie, J., Williams, K., Ruben, S., Felix, L. and Strang, J. (2003). Sentenced to treatment: early experience of drug treatment and testing orders in England. *European Addiction Research*, 9, 120–130.

Gossop, M., Marsden, J., Stewart, D. and Rolfe, A. (2000). Reductions in acquisitive crime and drug use after treatment of addiction problems: one-year follow-up outcomes. *Drug and Alcohol Dependence*, 58, 197–204.

Grapendaal, M. *et al.* (eds) (1994). Legalization, decriminalization and the reduction of crime. In E. Leuw and I. H. Marshall (eds) *Between Prohibition and Legalization. The Dutch experiment in drug policy*. Amsterdam and New York: Kugler.

Hubbard, R. L., Marsden, M. E., Rachal, J. A., Harwood, H. J., Cavanagh, E. R. and Ginzburg, H. M. (1989). *Drug Abuse Treatment: A national study of effectiveness*. Carey: University of North Carolina Press.

Kothari, G., Marsden, J. and Strang, J. (2002). Addiction treatment in co-ordination with the criminal justice system: the Drug Treatment and Testing Orders (DTTOs) in England. *British Journal of Criminology*, 42, 412–32.

Marsch, L. A. (1998). The efficacy of methadone maintenance interventions on reducing illicit opiate use, HIV risk behaviour, and criminality: a meta-analysis. *Addiction*, 93, 515–532.

Rotgers, F. (1992). Coercion in addictions treatment. *Annual Review of Addictions Research and Treatment*, 2, 403–415.

Sees, K. L. *et al.* (2000). Methadone maintenance vs 180 day psychosocially enriched detoxification for treatment of opioid dependence: a randomised controlled trial. *Journal of the American Medical Association (JAMA)*, 283, 1303–1310.

Simpson, D. D. (1990). Longitudinal outcome patterns. In D. D. Simpson and S. B. Sells (eds) *Opioid Addiction and Treatment: A 12 year follow-up*. Florida, USA: Robert E. Krieger.

Szasz, T. (1982). The war against drugs. *Journal of Drug Issues*, 12(1), 115–122.

Turnbull, P., McSweeney, T., Webster, R., Edmunds, M. and Hough, M. (2000). *Drug treatment and testing orders: final report*. Home Office, London.

Chapter 17

The Government Task Force and its review of drug treatment services

The promotion of an evidence-based approach

John Polkinghorne, Michael Gossop and John Strang

Background

The Task Force was set up in April 1994 on the initiative of a health minister of the time, Dr Brian Mawhinney. The terms of reference given to it were:

> To conduct a comprehensive survey of clinical, operational and cost effectiveness of existing services for drug misusers; to review current policy in relation to the principal objective of assisting drug misusers to achieve and maintain a drug free state, and the secondary objective of reducing harm caused to themselves and others by those who continue to use drugs; to make recommendations where appropriate and to report to Ministers.
>
> (Task Force Report 1996)

The Task Force was set up by the Department of Health in relation to services for whose provision it was directly responsible and hence its work only related explicitly to England, though the corresponding authorities in Scotland, Northern Ireland and Wales expressed clear interest in the outcomes of its work.

The background to the setting up of the Task Force undoubtedly included general anxiety at what was seen to be an increasing incidence of drug misuse in the United Kingdom, together with the feeling that something must be done about it. There were also more particular worries. One, which was included in the Task Force's terms of reference, was that treatment might often be insufficiently oriented towards the attainment of abstinence. More specifically in this connection, there were those who questioned the acceptability and legitimacy of methadone maintenance programmes, which seemed to some simply to replace an illegal drug with a similar drug legally prescribed. There was also concern at how well services were organised and coordinated, and anxiety about how well they were succeeding in being available to teenagers who needed their help.

From the outset, it was clear that the project was an extensive one and therefore the Task Force was given two years in which to complete its work. In this it succeeded and the Report was published on 1 May 1996. The Task Force was also giving a budget of a million pounds spread over the two years. The largeness of this sum stemmed from the recognition that the conclusions and recommendations of the Report needed to be evidentially based, and so the Task Force would need to commission a number of research projects to assist it in its thinking. These would require the availability of financial resources on a significant scale.

Making the Task Force work

In addition to its Chairman, the Task Force had 12 original members, three of whom left before the completion of the Report, and one new member joined in December 1994. They came from a variety of backgrounds, some with direct experience of drug treatment problems, some coming from more general health or community services settings, and some with no previous experience of drug matters at all. There was some criticism that no member of the Task Force was drawn from those who were engaged in service provision, or from the pharmacy profession. It was obviously not possible to represent directly every relevant speciality and the Task Force sought written and oral presentations from organisations and individuals with a wide range of experience and advice to offer. It also made a number of visits to centres and institutions where work could be observed. In total, it received 167 inputs of these various kinds, which were of considerable help and significance in its work.

The Chairman of the Task Force was the Reverend Dr John Polkinghorne, FRS, at the time the President of Queens' College, Cambridge. Polkinghorne summarised his own position, and the position of the Task Force, thus:

> I came to the work of the Task Force without any prior knowledge and experience of the problems of drug misuse. However, my scientific background (which is in theoretical physics) had accustomed me to the assessments of evidence-based beliefs. I had also had a good deal of experience of acting as a chairman who is seeking to find an acceptable consensus. This experience had included taking the chair of Department of Health committees that made recommendations to Ministers concerning social and ethical questions relating to aspects of medical practice. On joining the Task Force, I found myself on a steep learning curve. It was soon clear that the drug scene was one of great complexity in which it would not be possible to lay down a single procedure that could be universally relied on, or a simple goal that could be universally attained. It was rather a case of 'horses for courses', where different presenters would need different forms of response, and where the presence of both

progress and relapse implied that it would often be necessary, at least initially, to aim for limited but worthwhile gains. I was greatly helped in my responsibility by the willing cooperation and hard work of the members of the Task Force. We soon established mutual confidence in each other and we were able to able to act together as a team almost from the start. We also received indispensable support from our advisers.

(Polkinghorne 1995: 4)

Gathering and creating the missing evidence base

The Task Force soon resolved that a key feature of its eventual Report must be the careful evaluation of evidence on which its conclusions were to be based. It therefore set to work to gather appropriate information through consultations and through the research projects that it sponsored. As described below, the most substantial part of this exercise was the National Treatment Outcomes Research Study (NTORS).

The sorts of evidence that could be gathered by the Task Force varied with the kinds of question whose answer was being sought, and with the size of the sample that could be investigated. Although the research tried wherever possible to rise above the merely anecdotal, there was also a limited but legitimate role for the use of anecdote as a source of insight into the experience of individuals. In the case of some of the studies, the size of the available sample may not have been large enough to enable generalisation beyond well-based qualitative conclusions. Only in the case of studies with the largest sample sizes would it be possible to produce well-substantiated quantitative conclusions. Its budget allowed the Task Force to commission nine research projects, whose methodologies varied in accordance with what was appropriate for that particular investigation. These projects were all contracted out to suitable investigators. Their topics included the views of drug users on the services they had received; treatment of cocaine addiction; surveys of treatment systems and community-based agencies; services for young people; the role of community pharmacies and their dispensing of methadone; the training of drug workers; and an investigation of the course of drug addiction problems among an untreated sample of drug misusers.

The Task Force felt it appropriate to direct the major tranche of funding to NTORS. This was designed and directed by Prof. Michael Gossop at the National Addiction Centre at the Maudsley Hospital/Institute of Psychiatry. It was recognised at an early stage that a prospective study of this kind needed to continue well beyond the life of the Task Force and its budget, and it was a source of satisfaction to members of the Task Force that their recommendation that the financing of NTORS should continue was subsequently accepted.

NTORS investigated four major treatment modalities: specialist inpatient programmes; residential rehabilitation; methadone reduction programmes;

and methadone maintenance programmes. The four modalities were chosen because of their prominence in the portfolio of treatments actually being used within the UK, which also meant that samples could be recruited that were of sufficient size to enable the drawing of statistically significant conclusions. With the willing help of treatment providers, a cohort of more than a thousand participants was identified as they entered treatment and a procedure was set up to monitor them at regular intervals thereafter.

Another important source of information for the Task Force came from the reviews of particular topics that it was able to commission from international experts. In this way it sought to avoid 'reinventing the wheel' and it was able to benefit from accounts of global best practice.

The special contribution and legacy of NTORS

NTORS comprised a long-term prospective follow-up study of more than 1,000 drug users who entered one of the four types of treatment modality during a five-month period in 1995. Because of extreme time pressure, NTORS was conceived during 1994, began operation during the early months of 1995, and reported its preliminary findings to the Task Force in October 1995. These preliminary findings were necessarily confined to a detailed description of the patient group and the nature and severity of their presenting problems. The recommendations of the Task Force encouraged the Department of Health to provide further funding for the project which was extended to become a five-year longitudinal follow-up study. Paradoxically, the main and most interesting findings from NTORS only appeared after the Task Force itself had ceased to exist. However, the Task Force was still able to build upon some of the main themes of NTORS. One of these was the prioritisation of the study of the effectiveness of existing treatment programmes being delivered under day-to-day operating conditions. This was also a major issue for the American treatment outcome studies (such as DARP, TOPS and DATOS) upon which NTORS was largely modelled. In turn, NTORS has influenced others both nationally and internationally, and has encouraged the implementation of similar projects in Australia, Scotland and Ireland.

Many of the outcomes reported by NTORS provided clear evidence of substantial and important reductions in illicit drug problems (reduced frequency and quantity of drug use, increased rates of abstinence), and reduced injecting risk behaviours. These changes were accompanied by improved psychological and physical health, and by substantial reductions in criminal behaviour. However, not all outcomes were so positive. Even in a treatment cohort which showed such major treatment gains, in the four years after intake, there was a continuing mortality rate of about 1 per cent per year (six times higher than for an age-matched group in the general population). In addition, many clients were drinking heavily at intake and continued to drink heavily throughout the five-year follow-up period. NTORS recommended that drug treatment services should be modified to address this continuing problem of alcohol consumption. Nor can the NTORS results be seen as showing that *any* or *every* type of treatment works. There was marked variability across treatment programmes both in treatments provided and in outcomes achieved by clients.

These (and other) results from NTORS have been reported in peer-refereed scientific journals. They have also been presented to the treatment planners, service providers and their clinical staff through a series of Department of Health bulletins and in a major national conference held in Westminster in June 1999. NTORS has received the generally sympathetic and interested attention of policy makers, and was able to inform the development of UK treatment policy responses in several ways. In addition to its contribution to the Task Force's report to the British Government in May 1996, NTORS has also provided information used by the Department of Health to formulate guidance to treatment purchasers, and contributed to the Government's *Ten Year Strategy for Tackling Drug Misuse*.

The longer-term impact of NTORS and the Task Force

The impact of NTORS has turned out to be far wider and more diverse than was probably originally envisaged.

The main study findings and its conclusions have been generally well received by those working in British treatment programmes. This is not surprising since most results have been positive, and have been interpreted as supporting the 'treatment works' message. There was also a further and extremely interesting spin-off from the study. The manner in which the project was conducted and the results presented appears to have contributed towards what has been a significant change in the attitudes of clinical service providers towards the role and the value of treatment research. Earlier attitudes of cynicism and resistance have been largely supplanted by a greater willingness to embrace research as an ally and a supporter of the work of the addiction services.

One possibly unfortunate side effect of the influence of NTORS has been to encourage a greater focus upon reduced crime as a goal of drug misuse treatment services. NTORS hoped that its results would contribute to the debate about how best to allocate scarce economic resources to tackle drug misuse problems, and about the merit of retaining the current imbalance in resource allocation whereby the greatest economic commitment is to repression or other supply reduction measures rather than treatment. Subsequent to NTORS and the publication of the Task Force Report, although increased resources have been directed towards treatment, there has also been a very marked change of focus whereby crime reduction has moved to the top of the list of political and social priorities for drug misuse treatment.

Summary of outputs of the Task Force

The Report of the Task Force covered 146 pages and it made 79 recommendations. On publication, the relevant health minister, who by then was Mr John Bowis, stated that the Department would be studying the recommendations and that it would be drawing up guidance for health and local authorities, based on the findings. He also announced an immediate increase of funding, amounting to six million pounds, to be used to improve services for young people and to develop methadone programmes. Salient points made and conclusions reached in the Report included:

1   Drug misuse represents a complex and diverse scene, producing serious consequences both for the lives of misusers and for society generally. People tend to present to treatment services only after many years of drug misuse. By then their general state of health is often very poor. Drug misuse is a highly significant factor in the generation of crime. The 1,075 participants in NTORS stated that they had, in the three months prior to their admission to treatment, been involved in 70,000 criminal acts. The cost to society of these acts in the three-month period was estimated at approximately four to five million pounds.

2   A simple summary of the conclusions to be drawn from NTORS could be expressed in the slogan 'Treatment works'. Of course, this had to be understood in a careful and nuanced way. No 'magic bullet' had been identified that would lead simply and straightforwardly to the attainment of abstinence. Nevertheless, it had been demonstrated that treatment could produce significant and cost-effective reductions of the harm being done both to misusers and also to society. This was true of all the four modalities considered. Further study would be necessary if it were to prove possible to match clients and modalities most effectively.

3   In many cases the realistic expectation was of some form of step-by-step improvement. While abstinence is the ultimate aim, it is unlikely to be attainable at one leap. Small gains are better than no gains at all. Harm minimisation is highly desirable and the Task Force recommended a programme of universal vaccination of drug misusers against hepatitis B, and that general health checks should be made on clients on presentation. They also affirmed the value of syringe exchange schemes in relation to harm minimisation. For many opiate misusers, methadone reduction and methadone maintenance programmes were seen to have an important role to play in promoting stabilisation and functioning in society. Since an important gain is the move from injection to oral use,

the Task Force recommended restrictions on the prescription of injectable opiates and also that methadone should not be prescribed in the form of tablets that could readily be crushed and injected.

4   In a regime characterised by volatility of intention and by relapse, prompt response to presentation is essential. Monitoring of performance, both by purchasers and by providers, was seen as being important and the Task Force suggested a set of relevant performance indicators that could be used for this purpose. Counselling was recognised as being an important component in all treatments of drug misusers. It should be of a professional standard, clearly distinguished from general befriending.

5   Although specialist centres have an indispensable role to play in drug treatment, the Task Force recommended extended use of some GPs acting to give 'shared care' under the direction of such a centre. There was also encouragement for the exploration of the possibility of an enhanced role for some pharmacists. The many opportunities for contact with drug misusers offered by accident and emergency departments needed to be exploited appropriately.

6   Many drug misusers become involved with the criminal justice system and this can offer important opportunities for initiating treatment. The Task Force received evidence that legal requirement did not reduce the effectiveness of treatment. Taking full advantage of these opportunities would require that the standards of treatment available within the prison system should be comparable to those operating outside. It is extremely important also to ensure that prisoners receive continuity of care on their release from prison.

7   Meeting the social needs of drug misusers in relation to matters such as employment and accommodation, can play a very important part in facilitating the effectiveness of treatment and rehabilitation. The Task Force, therefore, emphasised the necessity for close cooperation between health and social services in meeting the whole needs of drug misusers. Effective treatment depends on dealing with both medical and social problems together.

8   The Task Force received evidence that teenage drug misusers were extremely reluctant to make use of available treatment facilities, because they felt this identified them in an unacceptable way with adult 'junkies'. Therefore, it recommended that special provision should be made to meet the needs of this age group.

Concluding observations

Just like politicians and rock stars, Government reports come and go. Usually they are largely forgotten within a year or two, withering away in historical archive stores. But some, such as the Task Force Report, are different. They were fresh and relevant at the time, and, perhaps more surprisingly, they again seem so when re-visited after their initial impact. More than eight years after its publication, the Task Force report remains relevant and the priorities identified within the report remain highly relevant to current issues for the drugs fields today. Some of the recommendations have been acted upon, with healthy improvement to drug services in the UK. But others have elicited only limp and half-hearted responses, or rhetoric with little accompanying change. A periodic re-visiting would be a wise and rewarding exercise.

References

Polkinghorne, J. (1995). The Department of Health's Task Force to review services for drug services. A progress report. *Druglink*, 10(1): 4 (suppl.).

Task Force to review services for drug misusers (1996). Report of an independent review of drug treatment services in England. London: Department of Health.

Chapter 18

The 'British System' of drug policy

Extraordinary individual freedom, but to what end?

John Strang and Michael Gossop

(This chapter draws subtantially on the chapter previously written by John Strang and Michael Gossop and published in the 1994 edition of *Heroin Addiction and Drug Policy*, Oxford University Press, supplemented by additional material from John Witton, Francis Keaney and John Strang in a chapter on the history of the British System, which appeared in the book on *Drug Misuse and Community Pharmacy*, edited by Janie Sheridan and John Strang and published in 2002 by Taylor & Francis.)

It has not been the way of things in the UK to construct formal drugs policy. Policy changes are often seen to have occurred only with the benefit of hindsight. Paradoxically, the most distinctive characteristic of the British System over the years may be the lack of any defining characteristic. Amongst the (probably unintended) benefits of this approach may be the avoidance of the pursuit of extreme solutions and hence an ability to tolerate imperfection, alongside a greater freedom, and hence a particular capacity for evolution.

There is certainly no explicit set of rules or central policy underpinning an organized system to which observed benefits can be attributed. So one might conclude that there is no point in any further examination of the British System. However, despite the lack of formal structure over the years, characteristics of a distinctive British approach can certainly be discerned, and there are particular components within the British responses which deserve special study. There may be no clear system; it may not be particularly British; but there may well be benefits to be accrued from an examination of policy in Britain – even if the policy has often been policy by default.

Looking back at Britain's national response to its drug problems during the twentieth century, it is almost impossible not also to look across the Atlantic and to make comparisons with US drug policy which has been so influential on the international scene. It is not only that US government expenditure on drug policy far exceeds UK expenditure, it is also that the governing ideas behind the different policies have often been remarkably different. This was evident during the early years of the twentieth century when the courses of British and US drug policy diverged with the passage of the 1914 Harrison Act (and the threat of prosecution in the years that followed) in the USA and the 1926 Rolleston Report in the UK. These differences have surfaced again recently with the British interest in identifying harm-reduction measures which are directed towards improving the well-being of the ongoing drug user. This harm-reduction approach stands in stark contrast to the 'zero tolerance option', 'user accountability', and the US goal of a 'drug free America' (Kleber 1993).

Much attention has been focused upon the differences between British and American approaches in the period between the 1920s and the 1960s, when the USA pursued a policy reliant solely on control measures. Over these years, the UK, with its much smaller injecting drug problem, pursued the path of medicalization of the condition of drug dependence, even though the Home Office used its influence to try to push Britain towards a system similar to that of the USA and a reliance upon an entirely penal approach with criminal sanctions against both users and prescribing doctors (Berridge 1984).

During the 1960s, both the UK and the USA re-examined and revised their policies. America 'discovered' methadone maintenance through the work of Dole and Nyswander, and methadone maintenance programmes were established. Such substitution programmes found acceptance from practitioners, politicians and the general public, on the basis that they represented a 'treatment' of the underlying 'disease' (the manifestations of which included social, economic and criminal disturbances). In the UK, a different re-examination was taking place, with the prescribing of drugs being seen as a 'bait' with which to 'capture' the addict into the treatment programme. The prescription of heroin or methadone was seen more as a pragmatic and instrumental measure and not in the same narrow 'treatment' light as in America. At the same time, US programmes developed in a more business-like manner and were largely constructed along the lines of public policy or public health measures, whereas UK treatment was still delivered in the paradigm of individual treatment negotiated between doctor and patient.

In the UK, a great deal of attention has been paid to the development of strategies which may lead the drug user into less harmful patterns of drug use – and many of these approaches have been covered by the broad term 'harm reduction'. Thus the provision of methadone is not seen as the treatment in itself but as part of a package which is designed to encourage the patient/client to approach and continue to attend the treatment service. In contrast, in the USA, the entirety of drug-taking behaviour is seen increasingly within an illness paradigm, which not only lends legitimacy to treatment measures and increases the likelihood of public and political support, but also leads to drug prescribing (such as methadone) being seen again as 'treatment', even though there is clear acknowledgement of the considerable extent to which the context of treatment delivery has such a considerable effect on the benefit of the treatment.

Policy and practice have certainly changed over the years. Whilst there are some points of change which relate to new legislation (such as the introduction of the new UK drug laws in 1967), a distinctive feature of the evolution of policy in the UK is that it has more often been achieved through the preparation of closet policy. For example, the Rolleston Committee, the Brain Committee, the Advisory Council on the Misuse of Drugs (ACMD) – these have all prepared recommendations for consideration by the Government through their special reports. Often these do not become official policy, but nevertheless they inform the process of development of services in the years that follow. Thus the 1982 'Treatment and Rehabilitation' Report from ACMD prompted the development of community services and community drug teams throughout the 1980s; and the 'AIDS and Drug Misuse' Reports from the ACMD (1988, 1989) played a similar role in relation to the new HIV-conscious drug services of the late 1980s and 1990s.

The different ages of the 'British System'

Perhaps with the benefit of that most useful of scientific devices, the retrospectoscope, it may be possible to discern certain distinct periods during which different variations of the 'British System' have been evident.

The Rolleston era

A relationship certainly existed between opium and the people long before the 1920s (cf. Berridge and Edwards 1981), but it was probably not until the publication of the Rolleston Report in 1926 (Departmental Committee on Morphine and Heroin Addiction) that a distinctly 'British System' can be identified. At a time when the early prescribing clinics in the USA had all been closed down, Britain was moving along an altogether different path, with opiate addiction becoming the legitimate domain of medical practice (and hence prescribing). As much as anything else, it is perhaps this contrast between the British and American paths which defines the British System of this time.

It is clear that the numbers of opiate addicts in the UK were extremely low during these years. Typically a few hundred cases came to official attention each year, of whom a substantial proportion were either health care professionals or 'therapeutic addicts' (a term used to describe individuals who became addicted to the drug during a period of therapeutic use – for pain relief, for example). What is far less certain is whether any causal relationship can be identified between the post-Rolleston British System and the absence of an opiate drug problem. Some commentators have confidently attributed many of the benefits to the policy and practice approaches of the day (for example, Schur 1966; Trebach 1982), whilst others have referred to this 'period of non-policy' (Smart 1984) or to a period during which 'there was no system, but as there was very little in the way of misuse of drugs, this did not matter' (Bewley 1975). Downes (1977) concluded that the British System had been 'well and truly exposed as little more than masterly inactivity in the face of what was an almost non-existent addiction problem'.

Crisis and review in the 1960s

With the migration of North American (mostly Canadian) injecting opiate addicts to the UK in the late 1950s and early 1960s, and with the emergence of a new and youthful drug-taking culture, the structural timbers of the old British System began to creak. Substantial numbers of young injecting drug takers began to be seen for the first time, and the existing British System was failing to limit the spread of this new pattern of heroin addiction, and actually appeared to be making matters worse. The second Brain Report (Interdepartmental Committee on Drug Addiction 1965) put forward three linked proposals – restrictions on the prescribing of heroin and cocaine, the establishment of drug treatment centres, and the introduction of the notification system. New guidelines from the Ministry of Health defined the role of the drug treatment centres as the provision of appropriate treatment to drug addicts, whilst also 'containing the spread of heroin addiction by continuing to supply this drug in minimum quantities where this is necessary in the opinion of the doctor; and where possible to persuade addicts to accept withdrawal treatment' (Ministry of Health 1967). Thus, as Stimson and Oppenheimer (1982) subsequently commented, the new treatment centres were given the twin responsibilities of medical care and social control.

In their early days, the new clinics prescribed injectable heroin in doses which were similar to the private prescribing doctors whom they replaced, although the average daily dose of prescribed heroin then fell steadily over the next few years. In their first flush of clinical practice, the clinics also prescribed injectable cocaine, but stopped this quite quickly within the first year of operation. Gradually, injectable forms of heroin were replaced by injectable methadone as the preferred drug of prescription (preferred by the clinic doctors, for whom injectable methadone was perhaps more closely aligned with treatment and could also be taken at less frequent intervals).

The original intention had been to draw all addicts into treatment, thereby containing the 'epidemic'. However, even during these early years of the clinics, there was evidence of a large population of drug users who remained out of contact with the new treatment centres. Blumberg *et al.* (1974) reported that, even by 1970/71, addicts attending the new treatment centres were reporting that only half of their drug-using friends were in treatment.

The middle years of the clinics: care or control?

The optimistic original view had been that, as a result of frequent contact with the new treatment centres, the drug user would be led to the realization that they should give up using drugs. However, in practice the effect of the regular contact and a secure supply of pharmaceutical injectable drugs often led to an institutionalization of drug use, with the addict becoming confirmed in their addiction, albeit a clinic-maintained addiction. As Edwards commented as early as 1969, 'the result of such a humane policy may sadly be the reverse of that intended: the drug taker is protected from all adverse social consequences of his addiction, and all motivation for withdrawal is sapped'. During the 1970s the clinic staff and especially the psychiatrists who were responsible for prescribing drugs lost enthusiasm – first for prescribing heroin and then for prescribing any injectable preparations (see Chapter 4, this volume). As the initial optimism was replaced by realism or even rebound pessimism, the London drug clinics appear to have undergone a collective existential crisis in the mid-1970s. Was their prime responsibility care of the individual patient, or the social control of addiction?

The hope that the prescribing of supplies of National Health Service injectable drugs would prevent the development of any black market appeared to be flawed, and was consequently largely abandoned – certainly at the broader policy level, although probably not at the individual level. Individual treatment or care came to be the dominant *raison d'être* of the drug treatment centres, whose work was increasingly managed by the multidisciplinary teams employed in the drug clinics. Oral methadone became the most commonly prescribed drug for new patients, and thus a therapeutic apartheid was created between small numbers of patients who had attended in the early years of the clinics (many of whom continued to receive injectable drugs) and the more recent addicts who were usually offered only oral methadone. It would appear that this combined shift in prescribing practice and the introduction of therapeutic contracts served to give disillusioned clinic staff a new sense of purpose and direction – perhaps with their energies being directed towards helping the drug addict to become abstinent.

Community-orientated services

A new community orientation to the delivery of care was introduced in the early 1980s, particularly following the publication of the Treatment and Rehabilitation Report from the ACMD (1982). Perhaps coinciding with the move away from prescribing as the focus for the intervention, and alongside a presumption that this prescribing would be of oral-only medication, the general practitioner was encouraged to be a readily available and local provider of care to the increasing numbers of heroin addicts in the community, many of whom had never had any contact with formal treatment services.

The era of the exclusive specialist was over. Provision of care to the drug user was now seen as part of the everyday work of all general practitioners (see Chapters 5 and 6, this volume). However, despite the central promotion of this model for at least a decade, the continued reluctance of many general practitioners remains evident. Whilst the gains which have been made represent a significant improvement in the local availability and provision of care, it is nevertheless still the case that many family doctors remain hostile to their proposed key involvement in looking after drug users – especially when this may involve the prescribing of substitute drugs such as methadone (see Chapter 7, this volume).

AIDS and the new HIV-conscious 'British System'

AIDS forced another fundamental re-examination of British drug policy, in which concerns about HIV and AIDS become the dominant public health issue. Injecting drug users (through their sharing of contaminated injecting equipment) were suddenly of special importance because they represented a potential 'bridgehead' for the spread of the virus – a potential route for HIV to diffuse rapidly into the wider community.

'Harm reduction strategies' came to the fore in this newly re-vitalized and re-orientated British System – through interventions aimed at the reduction of drug-related harm. In harm reduction strategies, the driving force is not the drug taking or abstinence of the drug user, but the extent to which harm has been reduced as a result of the intervention. This may occur at the level of harm for the individual, or harm for the broader population. Consideration of harm reduction interventions also requires an estimation of the likely course that the drug use would otherwise have followed, and must therefore be reviewed regularly – both for individuals and for systems.

The first UK governmental reaction came from Scotland – in the 1986 report from the Scottish Home and Health Department. This had been prompted by the discovery of a terrible undetected outbreak of HIV infection amongst injecting drug misusers in Edinburgh (see Chapter 10, Volume I). The resulting McClelland report (1986) introduced the concept of 'safer drug use' and proposed making sterile needles and syringes available to those who inject drugs. Improved treatment services and substitute prescribing were also seen as ways of reducing sharing levels and the spread of HIV infection. As with many other changes in British drug policy and practice over the years, the ease with which this change was introduced was helped considerably by the looseness of the existing legislation and regulations which defined the British System.

The introduction of needle exchange schemes did not require any new legislation to be passed, and did not even require a public government statement of support; rather, it just required the authorities to allow the spontaneous initiative to develop under its own impetus, supported or steered by a small project development grant here or an investigative study there. Instead of the need for an explicit declaration of political support, it was sufficient for there to be an absence of opposition from the civil servants and professional guardians of the 'System'. And so, from 1986 onwards, an increasing number of drug agencies began distributing syringes to injecting drug misusers – both to those already engaged in some form of treatment or on a waiting list for treatment and also, perhaps most controversially, to those with no wish for treatment whatsoever.

The 1988 ACMD report 'AIDS and Drug Misuse: Part 1' provided the template and rationale for a reorientation of drug treatment practice to meet the new challenge of drugs/HIV. The report stated that 'The spread of HIV is a greater threat to individual and public health than drug misuse. Accordingly, we believe that services which aim to minimize HIV risk behaviour by all available means should take precedence in development plans' (Advisory Council on the Misuse of Drugs 1988). Whilst reiterating that prescribing to drug users should still have an identified goal, the report advocated a hierarchy of treatment goals whose appropriateness depended on the user. The key aims were to attract seropositive drug misusers into treatment where they could be encouraged to stop using injecting equipment and to enable them to move away from injecting toward oral use (Strang 1990). Decreasing drug use and abstinence were further levels in the hierarchy. Harm minimization was consequently at the core of the policy and was receiving active support from the Government.

From the late 1980s onwards, harm minimization was embraced as a legitimate health policy objective, as well as representing a banner under which an increasing number of clinicians and agencies re-focused their energies and work (Strang and Farrell 1992; Stimson, 1990).

But whilst the prevalence rates for HIV amongst injecting drug users remains low, rates for hepatitis B and particularly hepatitis C are much higher and have presented a new challenge to treatment services (see Chapter 17, Volume I, by Tom Waller). And yet, as Tom Waller charts, the British system seems to be sleeping. With three-quarters of injecting drug misusers in some parts of the country already infected with hepatitis C, the long-term health implications of this silent epidemic are enormous. Public and professional anxiety about HIV led to a commendably prompt adaptation of the British System to this new threat. So why has the similar, and in some ways more real and pervasive, problem of hepatitis C elicited a response which is so far distinctly limp?

New guidelines for doctors – encouragement to prescribe or pressure to conform?

In order to encourage the generalist (i.e. non-addiction specialist) doctor to take a more active role in treating drug users, the Department of Health convened a Medical Working Group on Drug Dependence which produced *Guidelines of Good Clinical Practice in the Treatment of Drug Misuse* which were sent to all doctors in 1984. Later versions of the Guidelines (in 1991; and, most recently, in 1999) became more comprehensive in their scope and the range of practitioners to whom they were applicable, with the latest *Guidelines* being available in full to practitioners through the Internet (www.doh.gov.uk/drugs). These 1999 *Guidelines* appear to have been generally well-received by the broad mass of general practitioners (e.g. Keen 1999) and have prompted the establishment of a new scheme of addictions training for primary care practitioners, although it remains to be seen whether the proposed identification of different levels of expertise (the generalist; the specialised generalist; and the specialist) is accepted as the basis for a co-ordinated expansion of different forms of addiction treatment provision across the country. The role of the prescribing doctor is likely to be a contested area for some time to come.

The re-emergence of maintenance

In the light of the new public health reappraisal prompted by HIV, maintenance prescribing once again moved centre stage – on this occasion in the form of oral methadone maintenance. Over the previous couple of decades, an impressive body of evidence in support of oral methadone maintenance had been established (especially from the USA) which demonstrated its effectiveness at promoting, amongst other benefits, marked reductions in continued heroin use and continued injecting. In the new climate, the publication and wider presentation of reviews of this evidence (see Farrell *et al.*, 1994; Ward *et al.*, 1992; and Chapter 9, this volume) contributed to the wider acceptance in the UK of oral methadone maintenance as a central plank of the combined drug/HIV treatment response. Once the prerogative of the specialist drug clinics, methadone maintenance treatment is increasingly provided by general practitioners, either independently or in a 'shared care' scheme (see Chapters 6 and 7, this volume).

Even within the plans for wider provision of well-organized oral methadone maintenance (see Chapter 9, this volume), there is still uncertainty and confusion about how it should actually be delivered. One of the concrete illustrations of this uncertainty is around the importance, or otherwise, of supervised consumption of the prescribed methadone. On the one hand it is argued that the lack of supervision of consumption of prescribed methadone fails to foster good compliance and also leads to the growth of an illicit market in diverted methadone, directly responsible for several hundred deaths per year. On the other hand it is argued that intrusive demands for endless attendance at clinics or pharmacies for supervised consumption is an unnecessary intrusion into the lifestyle of the patient and an extravagant waste of scarce staff resources, and that it may even drive the drug user back to the illicit market. Sadly, in a way which illustrates one of the unimpressive features of the modern-day British system, this important subject is explored by invitation for different parties to express their opinions, likes and dislikes. Surely it should be possible to find the best way forward by looking at the substantial international experience (despite the very different contexts within which these other treatments will have been provided) and to identify the necessary serious investigations in the UK which are needed to establish the amount of benefit that results from this greater supervision, the number of lives saved, and the extent of disadvantage and deterrence from the treatment system. However, despite serious encouragement to become more evidence-based (see Chapter 17, this volume), local policy and practice in the UK continues to be largely determined by local popularity poll and the whim of key local decision-makers.

Continued uncertainty – prescribing heroin and other injectable drugs

In the light of the considerable media interest in the recent use of injectable heroin in addiction treatment programmes in Switzerland and Australia, the UK began to look at this area seriously once again in the late 1990s and the early part of the new century. Although legally permitted, it is rare for injectable maintenance to be used (see Chapter 1, this volume): in practice in today's British System, most practitioners do not take advantage of this clinical freedom that they have (and have, in fact, always had). By the mid-1990s, heroin formed only 1–2 per cent of all opiate prescriptions (Strang and Sheridan 1997), with a further 9 per cent being for injectable methadone (Strang et al. 1996). Thereafter this figure continued to decline so that, by 2002, injectable heroin comprised only 1 per cent and injectable methadone only 3 per cent of all opiate prescriptions in addiction treatment (Strang and Sheridan 2003).

There are no defined limits on the amount of injectable opiates that can be prescribed nor any agreed criteria for deciding which patients would be appropriate for such treatment. However, the 1999 Department of Health *Guidelines* made at least some preliminary steps towards defining the 'suitable case' as being only potentially suitable for those patients who have failed other forms of treatment. These patients are likely to have been injecting for a long time, to be at increased risk of overdosing and contracting blood-borne diseases and being involved in criminal activities. Recent small-scale studies in the UK have suggested that participants had made significant improvements in health, injecting behaviour and social functioning (Strang et al. 2000; Metrebian et al. 1998). The recent Cochrane review identified only three eligible trials of heroin maintenance – the Hartnoll et al. (1980) trial from the UK in the 1970s, the Perneger et al. (1998) trial from Switzerland in the 1990s, and the van den Brink (2003) trial from the

Netherlands in the last few years. And these latter two studies, with their new interpretation of the old 'British System' heroin maintenance treatment, have kick-started a new international consideration. Nevertheless, the UK evidence base to support the efficacy and safety of injectable opiate maintenance remains small and this has prompted calls for rigorous and well-designed research to improve the evidence for this aspect of the British system (Zador 2001; and see Chapter 10, this volume).

1990s: crime reduction to the fore

By the early 1990s it had become clear that the UK had not seen the major spread of HIV infection among injecting drug users that many had feared. However, the 'drug problem' remained high on the wider political agenda and new policy developments continued. With the growth of recreational drug use in the late 1980s and early 1990s, the Government published 'Tackling Drugs Together: a strategy for England 1995–1998', in which it sought to combine 'accessible treatment' with 'vigorous law enforcement . . . and a new emphasis on education and prevention'. The aim of the strategy was to try to address, simultaneously, two very different objectives – on the one hand to increase community safety from crime whilst also addressing the health risks and other damage related to drug use.

Over this same period, NTORS was reporting on the substantial interplay between heroin addiction and criminal behaviour (especially acquisitive crime such as property thefts). Amongst the widely-publicised findings from NTORS was the observation that opiate addiction treatment was associated with major reductions in criminal behaviour (Gossop et al. 1999, 2000; and see Chapter 17, this volume) – to such an extent that it was possible to calculate that each pound spent on treatment was associated with a three-pound reduction in the costs to society (largely as a result of reduced levels of acquisitive crime and associated costs of the criminal justice system). This finding became public at a time when the drug–crime link was already becoming the dominant political concern about drug misuse (having overtaken HIV and health concerns as the main driving force). As a result, a strange strategic alliance was formed between law enforcement and the call for greater access to treatment.

Treatment was thus re-conceptualized as an intervention which might lead to reduction of criminal behaviour. Drug-using criminals were to be encouraged to enter treatment as a means of altering their behaviour (and mitigating the sentence that otherwise would have been imposed). Policy initiatives and resources were introduced to link the criminal justice system and the treatment sector through DTTOs (Drug Treatment and Testing Orders) (see Chapter 16, this volume; and Kothari et al. 2002).

But, despite the political enthusiasm and the endorsements from police and journalists, it is not all plain sailing. Clinicians have expressed concern about the absurdity of a system which gives fast-track access to treatment for those drug users with court proceedings whilst leaving those drug users without court proceedings on a long waiting list. Such a system of therapeutic apartheid not only seems unjust, but also seems absurd. Surely there should be a more integrated way in which access to treatment could just be made more universally available (Finch *et al.* 2003). But maybe such a simple suggestion fails to understand one of the more unsavoury aspects of the British system – the extent to which treatment provision is not only driven by a motivation to provide treatment to this disenfranchised patient population, but is also driven by the wish of public bodies to address public anxieties about civil disorder and the wish of politicians to receive popular approval and votes. Look, for example, at the apparent political commitment to, and investment in, research of the pilot DTTO projects: at first glance, this would seem to be an impressive example of policy makers making appropriate use of the contribution of research to shaping the British System of the future. But look again (and look at Chapter 16, this volume, which offers a guide through this territory). This fuller second look reveals a more disappointing picture, with precious little evidence of the DTTO initiative being seriously appraised or modified in the light of the findings from the evaluation which, when examined dispassionately, do not properly match the ringing endorsement of the political soundbites that were being released.

Conclusion

So where does this all leave us in our exploration of the British System? On the one hand, it might appear that there is no special 'British System' – certainly no single 'British System'. However, there have been some distinctively British ways of addressing and dealing with the problems of drug use in society. Whether by the absence of a policy in any other direction, or by the identification of the covert policy document, the shape of the British System can be seen behind the responses to the changing drug problem in the UK. It is not a constant system, and its lack of tight definition is sometimes exasperating; but on occasions this same characteristic enables a more prompt response to changing circumstances (such as the advent of HIV, for example).

The first 80 years of the British System demonstrated the flexibility of the British approach and its ability to adapt to meet new challenges and policy demands – to help limit the impact of the illicit drug market in the 1960s and 1970s through to the reduction of the spread of HIV and AIDS in the 1990s. Many of the fundamental conflicts about the purpose of treatment and prescribing practice are still unresolved while tighter guidelines and the demands for higher treatment standards throughout health care further curb the prescribing doctor's freedom of manoeuvre.

One of the most significant omissions within the British System has been the failure to take advantage of the capacity of research to inform and guide national responses. Many questions that are centrally important to the national response could undoubtedly be stated in terms which permit empirical investigation. As such, the effectiveness of many components of the national response could have been (and still can be) investigated by properly designed research procedures. The reliance upon policy-by-committee or policy-by-default may sometimes work, but without research support it provides the most fallible and perilous foundation for an enterprise as momentous as the formulation and implementation of a national drugs policy.

Future policy under the British System may be determined either by changes in the process of overt or covert policy formation, or by the resolve not to pursue a different path. Whatever the mechanism of future policy formation, an appreciation of our recent and more distant past will increase the likelihood that we are able to preserve those features of the British System which we wish to preserve, whilst not being shackled to an old and inflexible framework of diverse policy products. At the end of the day, it may be that pragmatism and the capacity to change and respond to changing circumstances eventually prove themselves to be the most interesting, most enduring, and most distinctively British features of the British System.

References

ACMD (Advisory Council on the Misuse of Drugs) (1982). Treatment and rehabilitation. HMSO, London.

ACMD (1988). AIDS and drug misuse. Part 1. HMSO, London.

ACMD (1989). AIDS and drug misuse. Part 2. HMSO, London.

Berridge, V. (1984). Drugs and social policy: the establishment of drug control in Britain 1900–1930. *British Journal of Addiction*, 79, 17–29.

Berridge, V. and Edwards, G. (1981). *Opium and the people*. Penguin Books, Harmondsworth.

Bewley, T. H. (1975). Evaluation of addiction treatment in England. In *Drug dependence – treatment and treatment evaluation* (ed. H. Bostrom, T. Larsson and N. Ljungstedt), pp. 275–86. Almqvist & Wiksell International, Stockholm.

Blumberg, H. H., Cohen, S. D., Dronfield, B. F., Mordecai, E. A., Roberts, J. C. and Hawks, D. (1974). British opiate users: I – People approaching London drug treatment centres. *International Journal of the Addictions*, 9, 1–23.

Department of Health (1998). *Tackling drugs to build a better Britain: the government's ten-year strategy for tackling drugs misuse*. Department of Health, London.

Department of Health (1999). *Drug misuse and dependence – guidelines on clinical management*. Department of Health, London.

Department of Health and Social Security, Scotland (1986). HIV infection in drug abusers in Scotland. Department of Health and Social Security, Edinburgh.

Departmental Committee on Morphine and Heroin Addiction (1926). Report. (The Rolleston Report.) HMSO, London.

Downes, D. (1977). The drug addict as folk devil. In *Drugs and politics* (ed. P. Rock), pp. 89–97. Transaction Books, New Jersey.

Edwards, G. (1969). The British approach to the treatment of heroin addiction. *Lancet*, i, 768–72.

Farrell, M., Ward, J., Des Jarlais, D. C., Gossop, M., Stimson, G. V., Hall, W., Mattick, R. and Strang, J. (1994). Methadone maintenance programmes: review of new data with special reference to impact on HIV transmission. *British Medical Journal*, 309: 997–1001.

Finch, E., Brotchie, J., Williams, K., Ruben, S., Felix, L. and Strang, J. (2003). Sentenced to treatment: early experience of Drug Treatment and Testing Orders in England. *European Addiction Research*, 9, 131–7.

Gossop, M., Marsden, J., Stewart, D. and Rolfe, A. (1999). Treatment retention and one year outcomes for residential programmes in England. *Drug and Alcohol Dependence*, 57, 89–98.

Gossop, M., Marsden, J., Stewart, D. and Rolfe, A. (2000). Reductions in acquisitive crime and drug use after treatment of addiction problems: one year follow-up outcomes. *Drug and Alcohol Dependence*, 58, 165–72.

Hartnoll, R., Mitcheson, M., Battersby, A. *et al.* (1980). Evaluation of heroin maintenance in controlled trials. *Archives General Psychiatry*, 37, 877–83.

Interdepartmental Committee on Drug Addiction (1965). Second Report (Second Brain Report). HMSO, London.

Keen, J. (1999). Managing drug misusers in general practice: new Department of Health guidelines provide a benchmark of good practice. *British Medical Journal*, 318, 1503–4.

Kleber, H. (1993). The US anti-drug prevention strategy: science and policy connections. In *Drug, alcohol and tobacco: making the science and policy connections* (eds G. Edwards, J. Strang and J. Jaffe), pp. 109–20. Oxford University Press, Oxford.

Kothari, G., Marsden, J. and Strang, J. (2002). Opportunities and obstacles for effective treatment of drug misusers in the criminal justice system in England and Wales. *British Journal of Criminology*, 42, 412–32.

Metrebian, N., Shanahan, W., Wells, B. and Stimson, G. (1998). Feasibility of prescribing injectable heroin and methadone to opiate dependent drug users: associated health gains and harm reductions. *Medical Journal of Australia*, 168, 596–600.

Ministry of Health (1967). Treatment and supervision of heroin addiction, HM67/16. Ministry of Health, London.

Perneger, T. V., Giner, F., del Rio, M. and Mino, A. (1998). Pandomised trial of heroin maintenance programme for addicts who fail in conventional drug treatments. *British Medical Journal*, 317, 13–18.

Schur, E. M. (1966). *Narcotic addiction in Britain and America: the impact of public policy*. Associated Book Publishers, London.

Smart, C. (1984). Social policy and drug addiction: a critical study of policy development. *British Journal of Addiction*, 79, 31–9.

Stimson, G. V. (1990). AIDS and HIV: the challenge for British drug services. *British Journal of Addiction*, 85, 329–39.

Stimson, G. V. and Oppenheimer, E. (1982). *Heroin addiction: treatment and control in Britain*. Tavistock, London.

Strang, J. (1990). Intermediate goals and the process of change. In *AIDS and drug misuse* (eds J. Strang and G. Stimson). Routledge, London.

Strang, J. and Farrell, M. (1992). Harm Minimisation for drug users: when second best may be best first. *British Medical Journal*, 304: 1127–28.

Strang, J. and Sheridan, J. (1997). Heroin prescribing in the 'British System' of the mid-1990s: data from the 1995 national survey of community pharmacies in England and Wales. *Drug and Alcohol Review*, 16, 7–16.

Strang, J. and Sheridan, J. (2003). Effect of national guidelines on prescription of methadone: analysis of NHS prescription data, England 1990–2001. *British Medical Journal*, 327, 321–2.

Strang, J., Sheridan, J. and Barber, N. (1996). Prescribing injectable and oral methadone to opiate addicts: results from the 1995 national survey of community pharmacies in England and Wales. *British Medical Journal*, 313, 270–2.

Strang, J., Marsden, J., Cummins, M., Farrell, M., Finch, E., Gossop, M., Stewart, D. and Welch, S. (2000). Randomised trial of supervised injectable versus oral methadone maintenance: report on feasibility and six-month outcome. *Addiction*, 95, 1631–45.

Trebach, A. S. (1982). *The heroin solution*. Yale University Press, New Haven.

Van den Brink, W., Hendriks, V. M., Blanken, P., Koeter, M. W., van Zwieten, B. J. and van Ree, J. M. (2003). Medical prescription of heroin to treatment resistant heroin addicts: two randomized controlled trials. *British Medical Journal*, 327: 310.

Ward, J., Mattick, R. and Hall, W. (1992). *Key issues in methadone maintenance treatment*. University of New South Wales Press, Sydney.

Zador, D. (2001). Injectable opiate maintenance in the United Kingdom: is it good clinical practice? *Addiction*, 96, 547–53.

Index

Note: page numbers in Volume 1 in normal type, in Volume 2 in bold. Figures and tables in italics